Healing And Dealing

§§§

Essays On Becoming Wholed

Peter Cloud Panjoyah

ISBN: 978-1-9990631-1-5 (Audiobook)
       978-1-9990631-0-8 (Softcover)
       978-1-9990631-2-2 (E-Book)

Greenview Publishing
Hornby Island, BC
V0R 1Z0 CANADA

All poems and songs in this book were penned by the author unless otherwise noted.

Newborough font courtesy of Roger White

Cover art by Bee Wolf-Ray
http://instagram.com/beewolfray

Dedicated To
All Humanity

May We
Find Balance Now

Table of Contents

Preface

In 2001, living 4000 miles from New England where I grew up, I found myself talking across several months in email with my mother and sister about my take on the healing process, particularly my emotional healing journey. After many long backings and forthings, in which I would share a little about my process and they would ask questions about how I got there and what I got out of it, leading to more explication, I received feedback particularly from my sister Alison that I did a really good job explaining something that was in many cases quite esoteric and nonverbal, and that I should consider writing a book about it.

Meanwhile, I was four years into a new relationship with Bee Wolf-Ray, a woman who I've come to consider one of the clearest channels of spiritual information that I've ever heard. Bee would often "Be-Earth", a term she coined that she preferred to the notion or concept of channeling, holding forth on many aspects of healing from a deeper or greater aspect of her Self. We recorded many of these sessions, and I often transcribed them. Year after year since that time, she has brought forth many very helpful understandings and concepts that aided our own healing, information which comprised a significant portion of the raw material for this book, for which I am enormously grateful. We are still in partnership after twenty-three years and Bee is still BeEarthing helpful and impactful information to this day.

I absorbed and integrated much awareness along the way in receiving these BeEarthings from Bee that I felt could help others besides just the two of us in their own healing from trauma or simply life in western culture. In addition, I was heavily influenced by a series called "Right Use of Will" by Ceanne DeRohan, as well as, ultimately, what I grounded and integrated from my own source as a result of my personal growth process.

So in 2003 I decided to take the plunge and started penning monthly articles for my local newspaper which consisted of my take on aspects of the healing process. Bee was my editor and greatly assisted me each month in both illuminating and clarifying my points, helping prune my rough drafts down below the paper's word limit. I published some fifty articles across five years which were well received by my community. Somewhere during those five years I began expanding the articles' base material, fleshing out my topics and adding new ones, with the idea of taking up my sister's suggestion. You now hold the result in your hands (or have on your screen, as the case may be), after many delays, editing passes and self-publishing.

*   *   *   *   *   *   *   *

Introduction

For nearly thirty years I have been actively engaged in healing my own patterns and past. This process has consumed me, and I have been dedicated to and enchanted with it and all of its workings, both on the inner and the outer. I have also have studied the workings of energy at all levels and how that energy flow affects healing, taking years of classes and practicum, soon maintaining a private energy healing practice. In 1996, when I felt an inner urging to have this practice be more grounded in the physical, I began private study with various individual bodyworkers, and took several massage courses, revamping my healership into a massage practice that focused more on the physical and emotional aspects of healing, as opposed to the mental/spiritual aspects that occupied my time as an energy healer in the early to mid-90's.

Within these pages I offer some signposts outside conventional approaches to healing. I welcome disagreement, debate, and strong emotional response to what is said. My words are my opinions and my personal truth, not necessarily Truth, although opinions can sometimes be experienced as Truth if there is enough trust in their validity and practical applicability. What I offer has been time-tested in my own life, and in the lives of many of those in my healing community.

The recommendations and conclusions drawn in this book are off the beaten track and reflect a life currently being lived largely "off the grid". They are not intended to reinforce what you already know, but perhaps what you have suspected or conjectured. For example, many people have not realized that expressing emotions in sound could possibly be healing or a good thing; after all, won't we just create more of the same if we do that? Or could it be, like a pressure cooker being relieved of pent-up steam, that the dynamic, evolutionary creations we are become more functional and balanced if we hold less emotional charge?

This book is written in the hopes that it will help people think, feel and act upon changing and releasing old habits. It is divided into four parts across what I consider to be the four layers of the self: our "bottom line", the physical body; our inner feminine, the emotional body; our "halfway house" the mental body, and our eternal, timeless light of consciousness, the spiritual body, all of which comprise the Self as a whole. I include a fifth section which follows the first four, "The Relational Body: Love, Family, Friends and Others", for it is in this realm of life that the four bodies of our Self touch and interact with another's four.

Though the text is divided neatly into these five discrete sections, there is an emphasis and focus throughout on the issues of the emotional body and how to effectively deal with emotional triggers. I focus on the emotional body because this part of self seems to be in direst need, collectively speaking, of more evolved understanding. It has become abundantly clear to me that a deep inquiry into one's emotional backlog is not everybody's journey. But it *is* the work of some, and the beauty of finding out if you or someone you love are among the some is that, ultimately, healing is do-it-yourself work and has a self-selecting quality to it. That is, you try it and it works and you feel good about the process having an encouraging effect, or you ditch it if it seems or feels wrong for you. Or, you do not even try it because it does not draw you. Hopefully discarding such an inquiry is not rooted in a belief that might read, "I believe it works but it is just too hard and painful so I am going to give up and try a mental technique because it seems easier".

There are many suggestions for "healing and dealing" offered in this book. It may be tempting to believe a possible guilt message that if you don't apply all or most of the tips, healing and dealing is not for you, you have failed, or you are not a 'good' healer. Guilt, however, is not a truth teller. I encourage you to pick and choose what resonates for you to try on, and ditch the rest. Not every suggestion is meant for every person.

In addition, everyone has different pacing with their self-healing as unique individuals with unique right times, and cannot be compared lovingly to anyone else's healing path or arc of healing. Comparison energy is not in service to balancing and healing ourselves.

I have subtitled this book, "Essays on Becoming Wholed", because a dear friend said to me that, more than healing wounds, the impetus we all have towards "maximizing our potential" and recovering from what we have endured in all of our painful history is to become whole people again, to have access to *all* of our power, *all* of that great potential becoming actualized or well on its way, so that life becomes an exciting adventure again, in every single nook and cranny of our existence.

Healing is a process, and the process molds us, happens to us, takes us over in the best way possible, *becomes* us. Adding the 'd' onto the word 'whole' somehow indicates to me a progression; motion. Motion generated via the increasing energy of rising vibration, which happens when we express emotions and receive resultant understandings. Some people think of emotion, or e-motion, as shorthand for "energy in motion". All this considered, it feels right to coin the term "wholed" to more specifically reflect the ultimate outcome of the healing process.

I was not trying to reach every person with my columns, nor am I with this book. The kind of people I am hoping my words of encouragement might help are not those who have no apparent problems or ongoing issues in their lives. The kind of people I am trying to reach and perhaps help are the ones who are often having reversals in their fortunes, who "cannot win", who have seething cauldrons of old emotions in them that they are not sure how to deal with, or who may be having physical problems and wanting to reach for new ways of responding to them.

I feel it is important for people who read my words to know which category they fall into, by and large, so they know if the content is applicable to them or not. If it doesn't resonate, it simply means the material, or that part of the material, is not right for *you*. It may help to carry an awareness that different people on different paths need different help.

In describing examples or anecdotal illustrations of various healing scenarios, I often use the "third person feminine" convention of 'her', for several reasons. Firstly, it is too cumbersome to always use "him or her", secondly, third person masculine has gotten most of the airtime over the millennia and it is time for a balancing, and thirdly, especially when it comes to describing scenarios involving the emotional body, the feminine principle is what I most closely associate with emotionality.

At some point in the healing process many of us reach a point where we would like to have some sort of group or peer support. There are people all around us doing vulnerable, deep healing work. There are people doing this work that one can meet through the web, through various workshop communities, and through friends of friends. Intending to find them and staying open for opportunities to be with them will undoubtedly lead anyone who wants help from individuals and/or groups, to begin to develop the roots of a support system.

The words "healing and dealing" are sprinkled throughout the book. This phrase indicates the work that we do to clear ourselves of backed-up emotional charge and old habits of thought ("healing"), which in turn manifests an outward flow of action toward people and situations in our lives ("dealing") that reflect the dynamic balance we achieve, bit by bit, through consciously engaging in the process.

Healing and dealing is a reiterative process, like the fish that flops onto land only to slide back into the water twenty times before she grows legs and walks out for good. We make the same mistakes over and over again until we grow the legs of true depth of understanding and walk out of the sea of confusion and pattern. This is accomplished via the evolutionary process of the Wholing Selves We Are.

I wish you all good and strong healing and dealing. In so doing, may we reclaim ourselves in all our fullness and power, and bring balance back to life on Earth.

PCP
British Columbia
Spring 2020

* * * * * * * *

Part I

The Physical Body

Chapter 1: Tips For Long-Term Body Health

A Great Mixed Drink

I've been hearing about this great mixed drink. Unlike most mixed drinks, I hear the more you drink, the clearer you get. Heavy indulgence doesn't result in getting tanked or a crippling headache the next day. You don't have to wait in line at the liquor store to get some, and even minors can indulge freely. How do you make it? Two fingers hydrogen, one oxygen. Hey, barkeep, set my friends up over here...it's on me.

Make sure the glass stays full...as soon as you knock it back, top it off, as a visual cue for the next time you pass by your tankard, that there's more to be had. Guys, it's okay to chug-a-lug it like a triple shot. Drink and pee, drink and pee, all day long.

Feeling hungry a lot? Down a big glass, wait 15 minutes, and then see if you're really still hungry. We've grown so chronically thirsty for so long, we sometimes mistake our body's signal for more water as a call for food. For best results, drink a lot at room temperature on an empty stomach to give your body the highest high, and don't mix it with anything else -- juice is not the same thing. They don't call it a watering hole for nothing! Especially if you've just received bodywork, had a big cry, or have done a lot of physical activity. Flush those toxins!

Cooling Off Injuries

Then there's the frozen form of this elixir of life. Be cool. In fact, be cold. Get yourself one of those soft packs, wrap it in a hand towel, and put it on anything that hurts. Strap it on if it's going on a hard-to-balance place. Yeah, I know it feels better short-term if it's hot, but nothing brings that curative, long-term, deep secondary blood flow like ice. 10-15 minutes on...then take it off for another 10-15 minutes. Then on again, then off again. A total of three rounds, twice a day. Just chill those aches right out. Alternating cold with hot can be another successful experiment for your body, who speaks to you in a voice only *you* can hear. My body doesn't have the same needs as your body, which doesn't have the same needs as your friend's body, ad infinitum. This book isn't meant to be a bunch of one-size-fits-all techniques, it's more like a store – take what you need and leave the rest for someone else.

Breathe, Breathe In The Air

We live in a culture of shallow breathers. Shallow breathing starves the cells of our body and leads to all sorts of long-term nasties. You can go a few days without water, weeks without food, years without exercise but go a few minutes without oxygen and you will die. As far back as 1947 studies showed that normal cells can easily convert to cancer cells when chronically starved for oxygen. Lack of oxygen resulting from an overly rapid and shallow breath rate can contribute to heart disease, strokes, depression, sleep issues, fatigue, premature aging and nearly every malady known to humankind.

Corporate industry and the style of modern life, as well as its conveniences, have in many of us led to decreased outdoor activity and increased work indoors, coinciding with an increase in exposure to pollutants. Restrictive clothing such as tight waistbands, belts and bras compromises the ability to breathe fully and effortlessly and can contribute to digestive, elimination or lymphatic issues. These factors, combined with the subconscious fear of triggering the emotions stored in our body, help create shallow/rapid breathing patterns.

Cultivating an intent to face the emotions that can be stirred by continuous proper breathing allows one to begin the journey toward clearing the impediments to greater oxygen intake and resultant cellular health. When we intentionally breathe deeply, we stir the held fear, grief or anger in the rib cage and internal organs such as the lungs, heart, stomach, spleen and liver. This is a good thing if we have acceptance for the possible emotions that intentional deep breathing might surface.

Moving the lungs more fully with deeper breathing also assists in lymphatic fluid moving through the body. Only physical movement, including but not limited to deep breathing, can move lymphatic fluid through the glands and thereby eliminate wastes and toxins much more easily from the body. Besides physical movement, there is no other pump to keep your lymphatic fluid moving, as, for example, the heart is for the blood.

Oxygen

Oxygen is the key component in the production of ATP, the chemical basis of energy production in the body. Deeper, slower breathing increases production of ATP. Increased oxygenation also improves blood quality, aiding in the elimination of toxins. It especially improves overall brain function and pineal/pituitary gland rejuvenation. Skin becomes smoother and stress load on the heart is decreased (thanks in part to greater lung efficiency), resulting in lower blood pressure. Increased diaphragmatic range of motion "massages" the heart, liver, pancreas, stomach and small intestine, stimulating blood circulation in these organs.

Breaking Down A Deep Breath

The website http://holisticonline.com describes the "complete breath" in good detail. It starts with a "lower" breath inhalation that begins in the belly, and proceeds upward through a middle, intercostal breath (the lower ribcage expands to the side), completing the inhalation in an upper or high-ribcage chest expansion. Exhalation reverses this direction, and ends at the bottom of the exhale with a final component – what I call an inner hug, where the lower ribs give a gentle squeeze to the diaphragm. This squeeze not only eliminates the last bits of old air in the bottom of the lungs, but when the ribcage relaxes, the next breath begins automatically! This is where effortlessness can begin. Be in no rush to begin the next breath; pausing at the bottom of the breath for a few seconds brings its own benefits, particularly the resting of Body's systems. Although oxygen uptake occurs on the exhale and thus slow out-breath is recommended overall, sometimes my body likes to just "let go" the air all at once, without pushing. Allow Body to do either, just because you feel to in the moment. The lack of pushing or rushing into the next breath avoids hyperventilation as well.

If executed properly, this breathing style is effortless. Strain and deep breathing do not go together and will likely result in significant "forgetting" or a subtle giving-up by Body if you are pushing yourself. Practice and perseverance will help turn re-learning into a new integrated Body function with a huge upside.

To remind myself to breathe I made a bunch of coloured art focused around forms of the printed word "Breathe" and taped them up around my place. We need to breathe fully and deeply, as much as possible and create a newer, healthier habit for increasing our body's vitality in place of the one we were raised on: subconscious, shallow breathing. It's a process. You will forget many times a day to breathe fully. It's alright.

Diet

I am making a conscious decision to only include limited suggestions for diet in this book. The reason for this is that there are such varied needs for individual bodies at different phases and times of life, even day to day, that no suggested regimen for all people or even subgroups of people could possibly be appropriate. That said, I have a few general tips that may work for you if you try them out at different seasons of your life for various lengths of time. As noted, cultivating the art of checking in with and listening to Body is really the only way to know what is the right food or regimen for you at the right time.

No matter what suggested food regimen you try out, avoid zealotry or proselytizing your tried and true way, or intimating your way is the right way for another, for the reasons stated in the above paragraph.

Don't fight with your body's cravings; hold your intention to let an eating habit lapse and then if you give in to a craving, see what feelings arise, when you feel you can. Once momentum is gained and right time for the change arrives, a habit *falls away naturally*. You won't have to discipline it away.

One possibility to try is starting the day with a heavy intake of liquids such as herb tea with lemon, a green drink from powders or concentrates found in whole foods markets (heavily dilution is recommended to increase water intake, promoting toxin flush), freshly juiced fruits and veggies or a blended fruit'n'veggie smoothie. Conversely, other bodies require an influx of protein or carbs early in the day. Your body knows better than your mind, or my mind, what it wants.

However much you can moderate intake of wheat, dairy, sugar, alcohol, caffeine and refined/processed foods of all kinds can be helpful in keeping good balance and maintaining high chi levels.

Try working a raw meal or three into your diet every week. The benefits of a raw food diet are numerous and described in detail in many books and in many areas of interest on the internet, and again, are not appropriate for everyone at all times. Many people wax eloquently about the benefits of a 100% raw food diet on their health. Other humans with other body types, such as the vata body type in the Ayurvedic model, may find they need warm food, cooked or not.

A 100% raw diet may be particularly efficacious when dealing with life-threatening illnesses such as cancer or AIDS. Widespread research has indicated that bodies nourished on a diet of largely cooked meals are too acidic, and that an acidic pH within Body has been shown to be the root cause of nearly every illness or condition.

A raw foods diet has an alkalinizing effect on Body. It is recommended that a switch from a cooked-food diet to a raw food diet be accomplished gradually, slowly weaning Body away from cooked foods. If you ask, your body will let you know what it would like to try in terms of a regimen. Your body may require certain cooked foods in moderation, so checking in is crucial – every body's needs are unique.

Zealotry, whether individual or group, is a pattern in many societies. It is not healing and dealing, nor is it free will, to pressure or coerce another to eat how I do at any given time. Zealotry and its accompanying pressure of others will, with enough healing, give way to an acceptance of others' ways as right for them at a given time, even if not for me.

Stretching

Remember that stretching is a wonderful injury preventive for any type of physical exertion. Stretch shortly *after* you've begun to exercise. For example, on a long walk, be sure to stop and stretch any time you start to feel pain in a muscle or an area of your body. Stretching after exercise is just as important too. I like to keep moving during my stretches...in super slow motion. Keep in mind that holding stretches for too long can put an unnatural strain on the body.

Many people are into yoga, a discipline from which I too have received great benefit at certain times. Overall, my Body's preference is the do-it-yourself practice of Somatics, a low-impact Body meditation involving very slow movement that alternately contracts and extends muscle groups in order to release holding patterns within the body. Most major cities have a Hanna Somatics teacher offering weekend workshops to educate people of all ages on how to do these exercises. A few minutes of internet inquiry can lead you to your first exposure to this effective healing modality that can return muscular suppleness everywhere you want it. Elders in particular have found major success and ability to work with Somatics to release stored energy in their bodies, proving that nobody is "too old" to have vigorous, supple muscles and full use of their bodies.

Exercise, Movement and Inner Listening

Don't want to exercise? Don't "should" on yourself. Follow your body's urges as unconditionally as you can, and pay attention. Ask Body if s/he wants to go to that dance, or hike the mountain today. Ask, and listen inside. If the answer is no, follow that -- don't let your mind lead. Mind has led the way long enough. Body has rarely, if ever, been given the chance to lead! If the answer is yes, go for it. Every body's need is different, there *isn't* any "right way".

As always, when intending and moving toward balancing any part of the self, moderation is key. In addition to not pushing Body to work out if you really don't' feel like it, bodies are also made of muscle and muscles enjoy working, so giving Body a chance to move and exercise when desire is present keeps the heart healthy, muscles stimulated, lymphatic fluid moving and energy flowing. Over-disciplining or under-utilizing Body are extremes which do not serve the health of the whole Self.

Can't tell what your body wants, and feel frustrated with that? Accept that about yourself, that you can't hear clearly from your body right away, in that moment -- and ask again later.

Body Sovereignty

Most of us refer to Body as "my body", as if some master self in me "owns" my body, as if my body isn't really me but is somehow external to the "real" self, more like a vehicle to be maintained. "My" body doesn't like that...she's a sovereign, sentient, fully spiritual part of me with as much say-so and right to lead as mind or spirit. She is not a Toyota, she's a magical, loving, human ecosystem, made of Earth (a female)! Ask "your" body's name, see what you get, and play with that. Talk to her, ask what she wants. Ask her opinion. Include her in your decisions. You may be very surprised at what comes up in response.

Sleep Support

No sweetie to wrap yourself around at night? Or s/he doesn't like to cuddle during the dreamtime? Didn't know you could heal while sleeping? One healing answer is lots of pillows. Soft gooshy ones. For side sleeping, I like one pushed up against my back, right down to my tailbone. And one in front of me, to curl up with. And one between my knees. Or under my knees if I'm on my back, or under one raised hip if on my belly. All this allows joints and muscles to more fully relax and let go completely into that soft support, else butts, backs and shoulders wave in the night breeze causing muscles, tendons and ligaments to max out from having to work while the rest of you is off partying with Wynken, Blynken and Nod. And yes, that back-to-the-womb feeling one gets from all this pillow snuggling counts for a lot as well in the relaxation department.

Immune System Support

There are many natural/non-allopathic options and protocols for staying healthy, or when sick, speeding the onset of recovery. These include herbs and homeopathy. One's preferred modality can vary depending on the moment and what one is drawn to try. The strongest immunity booster I am aware of is Oil of Oregano. If Body calls for O of O, it's often three drops in a small glass of water, knocked back like a shot, two or three times a day. I sometimes combine this with a higher than usual intake of Vitamin C (1000mg an hour when trying to fend something off), and have experienced very good results. 50mg of zinc taken with a meal can boost immune response. Echinacea, taken three times a day for ten days, followed by two days' off, is a widely supported immune system helper as well.

My friend Siebrich reminds me that a cold shower will strengthen blood vessels and raise immunity in general. Even 30-45 seconds of cold at the end of a normal temperature shower can be effective.

Western Medicine vs. Self-Care

I haven't gone to see the doctor in over twenty-five years. Only once in the last twenty-five have I stepped inside a doctor's office for anything other than bone trauma. Lucky? Maybe. My avoidance of the Clinic has, I believe, more to do with stepping up to take responsibility for my own health and educating myself about non-allopathic alternatives.

We are trained to give the power for our health to our physician, asking him or her to fix us. To do so is not necessary, can be potentially damaging and can limit, disrupt or completely sublimate Body's natural healing cycle. We are not taught in our schools that this cycle even exists.

Traditional medical "healing" options such as drugs and surgery nearly universally treat symptoms, not root causes, and the potential for deep, lasting healing is masked by a quick fix or Body-numbing drugs. Moreover, the profit-driven nature of pharmaceutical and surgical medical solutions presents a conflict of interest when it comes to doing what is best for Body.

Asking for help isn't wrong, it's definitely okay to reach for help, as sometimes bodies need help. When there is a broken bone or physical trauma from an accident, medical technology and skill is a welcome boon.

Ode To My Body

Body dear
    is what's the Matter here
Surprised that I fear
    And feel you
        So very very near

Heart here cries out
    In the scare
Of not being able
    To serve you

O yes, serve You
    Let you lead
Stop making you
    My worker steed
Want and wish and need
    To call home reversed love
In lives which yonder bleed
    Life force I need
On the uncaring sneering floors
    How life outside me deplores you!
Calls you a useless weed
    To be plucked and tossed aside
And lives ago I drowned in my pride
    Made you slink away

Finally... finally! Today
     I could notice what I'd done
Once removed you from my sun
     Sentenced you to cold and bitter ones;
Lost in barren warrens far from fun
     Wrong-made and forgot

Fortuitously, a plot
     Weaved by One not
So very far removed from who you are
     Who bades me go far
To recover you who I'd sent to war
     For surely "I" did not want to go
And in my sleep let you be G.I. Joe
     But somehow, t'weren't too late
To notice all my long-lost hate
     Which home converts to love.

O, once perverted dove
     Dive down deep into restful sleep
And bid today adieu
     Your bed is made anew
May your stay be comforting
     To the self so scorned for so long
Such a stuttering song
     You've flown many a far furlong
Now you can follow along
     As this Body flies and
Moves and grooves to the
     Fancied fetter-free future far-flung.

Chapter 2: Bodywork

Being a massage practitioner by trade, I'm a firm believer in healing touch. Get yourself some bodywork as soon as you feel you can. It's as crucial as anything else you might do for your body. There are likely many modalities of healing touch where you live, from massage to Reiki to Shiatsu to Feldenkrais Awareness to Reflexology, Somatics (see Ch. 6), Thai massage and beyond, available from many wonderful, loving and experienced practitioners. Talk to five friends, and you are bound to get a practitioner recommendation, either first or second-hand.

Bodies need to be touched -- loving, safe, healing touch. Touch is as important as breathing or exercising. Being touched with healing, honoring intent encourages the body to thrive and want to live, and live fully. Being touched aids in warding off depression and is a wonderful preventive for the dis-ease and dis-comfort that untouched bodies sooner or later manifest.

The Logistics Of Booking A Massage

No spare cash, you say? If you need and desire bodywork, you will find it one way or another. It may require some discipline, but setting aside some discretionary cash that you'd normally spend on other things can work. Everyone has something to offer – daring to suggest a full or partial barter with a professional or non-professional practitioner with willingness to persevere if the first attempt is rebuffed can result in a workable scenario.

Some bodyworkers are open to partial payment combined with partial barter, or time payments with a stated end time. Some are willing to use a sliding scale for their financially challenged clientele, and asking for what you need can be the key to expanding your options. Not every situation will meet your needs, but keep trying. Your intent to get the healing touch you need will pay off in right timing, even if money is an issue.

How to decide who to contact is another issue, especially if you've never met the practitioners in your area. Screening them via some questions over the phone can be helpful – the bodyworker's rates, the specialties they offer, how they respond if you present a particular ailment you'd like to bring into a proposed session, how they feel to you on an intuitive or subtle level are all important considerations. The experience level of the practitioner, while usually important, is not necessarily as crucial as how they feel to you up front or how sparkling the reviews are from someone you know and trust who has utilized their services in the past.

S l o w i n g Down

The ideal pace for the body to receive healing touch is very slow. Bodies can move quickly, yet speedy physical movement can be a sign that one is in one's head. Slow delivery of bodywork can literally allow greater embodiment for the receiver, bringing tangible contrast to her usual pace of life by encouraging her to slow down and merge with her physical self. Chronically moving too quickly can convey a sense of rushed anxiety and even contribute to injury. This can become a self-perpetuating cycle.

The massage table is a perfect place for Body to cycle down and become re-impressed with the health benefits of deliberate movement. Ideally, a healing touch practitioner aids this slowing down process with an unhurried application of the hands. Don't let guilt, caretaking, or habit prevent you from switching practitioners, even if the relationship is long-term, if your practitioner does not help you slow the pace of your life (or for any reason at all).

Suggestions for Receiving Massage

Becoming a good receiver is crucial to maximizing the pleasure and health benefits of bodywork. No matter what modality, an optimal bodywork session is one in which you (the client) are loosely, non-mentally focused and aware inside your body, particularly allowing that loose focus to rest upon the part of your body being touched at the moment, while maintaining a background awareness of how the rest of you is responding.

To facilitate this "locus of focus", talking should be kept to a minimum and should be centered on moment-to-moment needs and requests. Feel free to make lots of those! A bodywork session is a time to allow all your immediate physical needs to be addressed. A good practitioner welcomes your petitions for water, kleenex, a lighter touch, or another moment or two on that foot. If your practitioner initiates conversation and you notice that you are not as able to stay present in your body because of it, let them know that you are finding conversation distracting. If they persist, make that session your last with that person. A bodywork practitioner must aid you in becoming more embodied, not keep you in your head.

Do you find yourself endlessly spinning thoughts and visions during your session? This tends to occur organically, as bodywork connects the mind, spirit, emotions and body more efficiently than usual, and therefore, visions and possible solutions to issues in one's life can become spontaneously clear during a massage. Blood flow is increased. The stimulation of Body's self-healing response during massage reception is a demonstration of the magic of this kind of bodywork. As best you can, remind yourself that you can pursue that picture of the ideal job possibility or work through that tough issue with your spouse *after* your treatment, and return your awareness to your body, breathing deeply.

Slow, effortless breathing, especially extending the exhalation/outbreath, aids in muscle relaxation and is most called for during deep tissue massage of a particularly tight or painful muscle. This can be most efficacious by imagining you are located *inside* the muscle being currently worked, then breathing "through" that muscle slowly, deeply and as effortlessly as possible, as though there was a mouth on that spot inhaling and exhaling. On the exhale, it helps to consciously "let go" of the tension on that spot as it gets worked by the practitioner; in other words, surrender that tension to the touch on a physical level, allowing the muscle to relax as deeply as possible as you breathe out. Let the breath simply fall out of you, do not push it out, and do not be too hasty in reaching for the next inhalation. In other moments, it may feel best to simply let go of managing the breath in any way and allow a completely organic breathing response.

Most bodyworkers will encourage their clients to let them know if they are working too deeply or painfully on a particular muscle. Even if you as client are not reminded of this, it's important to take responsibility for yourself as a receiver and let your practitioner know simply and effectively when it hurts too much, with a short phrase such as "that's too deep", "too much right there", or "stop". Simply saying 'ouch, that hurts' may not get the message across to a practitioner who applies the 'no pain, no gain' maxim to a massage session, so be specific. The line gets crossed into 'too much' when it feels like you are fighting with the pain in order to withstand the current pressure, or you find yourself leaving your body when the pain increases suddenly as a given muscle is being worked, or noticing you are not wanting to "bother" your bodyworker with your "complaints" if the pain feels sudden and acute. Receiving deep tissue work is not a game of "how much can you stand" – that approach does not benefit Body.

This is not the time to hold back – your mental awareness can aid your body to stay balanced by speaking up when any of these conditions are not satisfied. A practitioner does not always know every single time s/he goes over a line into too much pressure on a given hotspot and requires your moment-to-moment feedback if you have any, so your body's needs can be best served.

My first masseur (the masculine form of the popular but often inappropriately applied feminine form 'masseuse') back in the late 80's gave me a guideline that I continue to repeat to my clients to this day: "Never help the practitioner". Raising your head or your legs to aid in pillow adjustment is a no-no. In a worst-case scenario, just-released muscles may go into spasm worse than before from being compelled from a state of deep relaxation to one of sudden contraction, simply from trying to help. Become "heavy- limbed" and allow the practitioner to move your body parts for you. Surrendering control of your body for the length of the session is a good habit to cultivate.

What does becoming heavy-limbed mean? It means giving full weight of your limb – i.e. dead weight – to the practitioner as they manipulate your limb for you. Imagining oneself as unable to move can help, as though you are a rag-doll for the time being. Deep, slow breathing is a key to surrendering control to the practitioner. Noticing what comes up for you in allowing this can be very educational; some of us have previous trauma in our lives that can be triggered by letting go of muscular control for even a few moments.

Emotional or Sexual Responses During Massage

Sometimes a bodywork session will stir old emotions as a result of a particular area being touched, rocked, massaged or otherwise manipulated. Allowing these triggers to rise to consciousness and dealing with them on the spot can be ultimately helpful. Again, holding back in this case is counter to healing. I recommend taking advantage of these "body triggers" by fully allowing vocal, non-verbal expression in moans, sighs, yells, cries, tears, and involuntary jerking (also known as kriyas). A sensitive practitioner will ride this wave with you, compassionately yet matter-of-factly supporting you in those moments. If this is not the case, you have another reason to switch practitioners.

Nearly every recipient of non-sexual, healing touch finds her or himself experiencing a sexual response at some point during any given session. This can be embarrassing or confusing, but such a physical response is perfectly normal. Significant sexual energy is stored in hips, buttocks and legs and can spontaneously begin to flow during a session when those areas are addressed. If this happens to you, continue to breathe deeply, stay in your body, and allow your response to run its course without action or comment. The responsible practitioner will do likewise.

Massage Aftercare

For the remainder of the day in which you receive a massage, take it easy. Errands and physical tasks are best left for another day. Let yourself move slowly, continuing the integration process of the massage. Drink more water than you think you need, to assist the body in cleansing toxins loosened by the massage.

Massage works deeply into the tissues and the cellular structure of the body. As our body is the storehouse for old emotions and pain, it isn't unusual for emotions to swim up later that day or even a day or two hence. Allowing these emotions to surface and dealing with them appropriately is part of your session overall. Body's self-healing mechanism is enhanced by massage, one of the great benefits of receiving.

Rotating Bodyworkers

Rotating bodyworkers can, in the long run, maximize healing for every part of your physical and emotional bodies. My own experiences receiving massage have reaffirmed for me that every bodyworker has specific strengths that work for particular parts of my body, but no one has the whole thing down. For example, where one person I see does wonders for my legs and hips, another affords my upper back and neck just the right pressure and motion to encourage maximum healing.

We tend to stay with one practitioner because they do good work overall, and there is nothing wrong with that approach. Yet, when I try a session from another practitioner, I find that certain areas of the body get addressed in new and different ways. It's important to put the body's overall needs ahead of long-term habit patterns.

Chapter 3: Habit Your Way

"Old habits die hard..." "We are creatures of habit..." "I am prey to my habits". Ah, the judgments we trot out in support of the same old same old. Even the contemplation of change can be a challenge, but we really set ourselves up when we equate ourselves to robotic victims of patterns that we expect we do not have the capability to shift, and therefore cannot muster the desire to try. Dropping the defeatist self-talk, we can begin to acknowledge ourselves as powerful captains of the ships of our own lives, with the wherewithal to manifest a sea change towards a more realized version of ourselves.

Habits Versus Addictions

Habits and addictions are related, but they are not quite the same thing. Where an addiction is often a substitute activity for what we really need (love, light, vitality, emotional freedom), a habit is more of an umbrella concept that includes any addiction, any kind of daily routine or any patterned behaviour that regularly repeats without us contemplating whether it is right time in this moment to enact this particular routine.

Routine can be a good thing and can be very comforting. Routine, at best, can help encourage the shifts in our lives by establishing familiarity. Yet when it comes to habits that are not serving us anymore, engaging in these habits is at that point an attempt to reproduce or recreate the memory of feeling good. Most often habits don't generate the same level of pleasure the habitual activity produced at an earlier time.

Habit patterns can include strung-together activities such as making coffee first thing in the morning, followed by turning on the computer and checking email, followed by rolling and smoking a cigarette, followed by a trip to the store. The majority of an entire day, weeks, or even years can transpire in similar chains of grooved activity. At these times, we are on automatic pilot, and we are not checking in with ourselves. Gradually Body loses the will to live, since She is not being consulted in the moment about what She'd like to do right now. As a result, illness can begin to manifest.

What Does Body Want Now?

Disciplining myself to change the habit without deep understanding of what was fueling it will likely only result in the habit changing form, say, from being on the computer first thing every morning to exercise. The goal is not to replace an old habit with another habit that is deemed healthier, but to be able to listen to Body's wisdom about what She wants to do in each moment. Sometimes when I am entering a period of free time I will intentionally imagine several scenarios that I might engage in now, and then check in with Body to see what I feel like doing the most, right now, be it what (or whether) to eat, or what to do. At my best, I might not allow my mind/spirit to imagine first, but simply invite Body's wisdom to present me a picture of what She would like to engage in.

There are often emotions hidden beneath the habit that the routine has helped me avoid, that can only be entered into when I allow the habit to lapse in order to see what is running beneath the routine. A crucial element in shifting the roots of habit patterns (without merely changing the form of the habit) is gaining understanding as to why I am engaging in the habitual behaviour, whatever that behaviour is, and often I need to clear emotional backlog hidden under the habit in order to truly get why I engage in the habit in the first place.

At most times, it's best to not try too hard to 'change', ourselves. This can also become a dangerous, unhealthy habit rooted in self-hatred. I have felt most relief in accepting myself as I am with all my addictions and habits. The root of all my unconscious behaviours is rooted in blocked emotions. By devoting myself to healing past trauma and emotional backlog, my habits and patterns change as I go, naturally.

Chapter 4: Fasting Down

The breakneck pace of summer in a tourist economy, or anywhere where speed of life can mean slipping unconsciously into ways of eating that don't serve me, requires a balancing time of reckoning for Body. Breaking old consumption habits is a wonderful way to cool down the pace, enhancing my life and helping me feel good about myself.

Fasting is not for everyone, so it's best to ask Body how it feels about trying one. Some folks never fast but do balance their eating lifestyle with taking breaks from substances for a while, such as sugar, coffee, dairy, processed foods, high starch grains, etc.

For those who feel good about trying it, fasting can give Body a much-needed break from the constant work of digestion, and helps initiate a cleanse of the entire digestive tract. There's nothing like a fast to break up embedded daily routine (what will you do with all that extra time normally spent shopping, cooking and eating?), dissolve cravings, and court epiphany. Fasting brings periods of detoxification for Body (including mental fuzziness) as well as periods of euphoria and great clarity and energy.

There is no "right way" to fast. Simply going without food for a number of days will help to give Body a break from all the digestion energy she normally expends. Some people fast using supplements and lower bowel tonics, others drink copious amounts of water and diluted fruit juice. Master Cleanser, aka "hippie whiskey" is a popular fasting aid, composed of a blend of water, lemon juice, cayenne and a dollop of maple syrup, ingested quart by quart.

Try taking a spoonful of psyllium husk twice a day during the fast in a large glass of water. This will help avoid constipation. There are other methods that can be researched of keeping the bowels flowing smoothly without food as well. Whether you choose a fasting/cleansing routine or simply listen closely to what your body wants to do in each moment, heavy liquid intake is a key component in helping cleanse the digestive tract.

Ritually entering a fast helps build and strengthen intention. The new moon, particularly a fire or earth moon (especially Virgo) is a wonderful time to begin, constituting an energetic clearing of the decks and the beginning of a new cycle. It can help to bring other types of intentions to such a ritual, such as intentions for change, healing, or new gifts and desires to manifest in your life. I prefer to fast sometime in the fall and/or in the spring; the extremes of temperature and energy output don't seem to call for Body to fast in summer or winter.

It is every Body's choice, moment by moment, as to how long to fast...even a day of fasting can help, though I like a three day minimum. I know of folks who've done month-long fasts and felt great. However long you choose, when re-feeding time is nigh, introduce foods minimally and gradually build up in volume over the first few days. Notice how your mouth has been re-sensitized (and how desensitized it had gotten just previous to the fast!). It's a great time to set a new baseline of eating slowly and mindfully, paying close attention to when we've had enough, including Body in our food choices, and becoming more aware of how we take in nourishment.

fffffFast

Fast…but it feels slow inside
        Tried to stem the tide, but
                no go
        Thick pudding brain with a citrus finish
What will I find that
        I once did hide,
shoveling down a landslide
        in imbalanced cry
                for help to fill the empty space,
or cover up the mess
        and relieve distress
                with a burp and a bellyful
So now I expect an exciting ride,
        tearing down the walls
                Of the habits denied;
the ones that say
        'we're just trying to live here…never fear'
So what's on the other side?
        Powers? Darkness? Demons? Hardness?
Perched on the precipice, it's hard to see
        what other facets I will find of me
I've jumped now, but only starting to fall,
        free flying thru a never-never land
Surely God will lend a hand,
        helping hoist the heavy heft
                that I've hurt myself with here
So I give me three cheers
        for hearing the scary unfelt fears
                call to me from under the plate,
                        for daring the hairy
                                food-free state
For untold days I'm choosing to wait,
        and my cup will run over
I'll liquidly sate

the hungry darkness --
We've got a date!

Chapter 5: Balancing Bodies and Computers

Personal computers enhance our lives in many ways, offering us convenience, ease of networking, socializing, commercial and creative advantage. Lots of home computers means lots of people often sitting in one position for lengthy periods. Balance being the key to a healthy lifestyle, we need to proactively take steps to counter this additional sedentary factor.

There are some easy ways to heal and deal around the uneasy marriage of body and computer. Stiff shoulders and necks are a major issue among computer users, especially in the trapezius muscle. Chronic tension in this area can lead to calcification, or the building of bone tissue in the muscle, which can lead to a multitude of problems.

Suggestions: **1) Type with your hands low.** Your hands on the keyboard should be no higher than navel level; any higher forces your shoulders to stay poised above their lowest possible resting point, creating unnecessary tension at the top of the shoulder blade. Stay aware of what the lowest resting point is, and either use a shorter table, pillows to raise yourself up, or a taller chair.

2) Take regular breaks to practice Somatics-style raising and lowering of the shoulders. By "Somatics-style" I mean super-slo-mo raising and lowering of the shoulders, starting at the bottom of the lowest resting point of the shoulders and very gradually raising your shoulders as high as they will go (up around your ears), then very gradually lowering them to the lowest resting point again. Repeat this motion several times, the slower the better, paying attention internally to which muscles are relaxing, which are working. Remember to breathe.

3) Undulate in your chair from time to time. I know this sounds weird, but try it... move from your trunk and at all your joints, all at the same time; for greatest benefit, move as slowly as you can. Bodies need to move often to stay happy.

4) Get up at least once every 30 minutes to move around. Stretch arms and legs even if it doesn't feel like you need to.

5) Get regular bodywork.

Other Office Detriments to Body

Many white-collar work environments such as offices focus on Mind and are not supportive of Body. Sunlight is often shut out. As much as possible, do not rely on interior lighting during the day, but supply Body with as much natural lighting as possible. Fluorescent or LED lighting is often the norm in office environments, and the vibration from these kinds of lights zaps Body's vitality. I recommend unscrewing overhead lights above your workstation and using indirect lamplight if no source of natural light is available where you normally sit to work.

Chairs purporting to be ergonomically helpful to body often put stress in new places such as knees when the lower back is supported. Modern office chairs tend to force Body into a position that may not be best for her in the long run. A straight-backed chair with a pillow supporting the lower back can be a healthy solution, where the pillow can be removed as necessary when body wants a break from that position.

Air quality is often stagnant in the office – take walks and get outside during the workday as much as possible.

For The Men

Sitting a lot in an office-style or any chair for that matter can accelerate prostatic stress. Nearly all men run into prostate issues at one point or another, and not just the elders among us. Notice the flow of your pee; is it strong from start to finish? If not, or if you seem to have the urge to go a lot even if you're not drinking many fluids, it's time to deal.

For the full-meal-deal, locate on your body what the ancient Chinese referred to as "the million dollar point", or the soft tissue just underneath and adjacent to your anus. While lying flat on your back, reach underneath your butt with one hand and put the middle and ring fingers against this point, using your body weight to allow yourself to sink onto your fingers, as deeply as you can without it hurting. Rotate your fingers three times clockwise, then the same counterclockwise, repeat both directions about five times, then switch hands for comfort and do it all again. If it's easier, you can stand up and perform the move that way.

This is a do-it-yourself prostate massage, a great proactive tool for keeping your prostate healthy, disgorging any trapped fluid buildup in the gland. This is best accomplished with pants on, jeans being the exception.

Other ways to support a healthy prostate: kegel-style pelvic floor squeezes, again best done slowly. Ask a mother what kegels are! Basically, you are slowly tightening your perineum, then letting it relax, also slowly. This can be done while sitting or standing. Also try occasionally and intentionally squeezing off the flow of pee. Be moderate with wheat, refined sugars, alcohol and caffeine.

Chapter 6: Body Meditations

There are ways to bring our conscious awareness more fully into our bodies, something even the more grounded among us probably need to do. Slow contraction and extension of the musculature is a good way to do this, and there are several forms of doing this. All forms involve breathing more deeply than usual. When Spirit and Body come into closer contact, blood pressure and stress can stabilize.

Somatics

Developed by Thomas Hanna in the 70s and taught today from the Novato Institute For Somatic Research and Training (http://somaticsed.com) and by certified practitioners worldwide, Somatics is one of the least known yet most effective ways I have found to drop deeply into my body and unlock holding patterns I was unaware of. It is a lower impact practice than yoga and is at least as effective.

Somatics works by isolating large muscle-mass areas of the body and, in super slow motion, gradually tightening them, then allowing them to fully extend and relax. The more slowly these exercises are done, the more effective.

When Somatics begins to unlock muscles in "sensory motor amnesia" (SMA is the state when muscles forget how to unwind and extend but remain in an unconscious clench) trapped energy there wants to come to life and vibrate after being held still for so long. This can be allowed via jaw chattering, grunts, sounds of all kinds, deep coughing and kriyas (i.e. spontaneous jerking movements the body makes when trapped energy is awakening, if allowed). There does not have to be a story to go along with any of this expression. I have seen this modality, when practiced along with the reception of regular bodywork, unlock lifelong holding patterns in the musculo-skeletal system that few other practices can accomplish, if any.

It is not expensive to be trained in the basics of Somatics as a do-it-yourself practice – one doesn't have to enter the four year program at the Novato Institute in order to have a working, applicable knowledge of the practice. To find a practitioner in your area who can teach you individually or within a weekend workshop style setting, surf out to:

http://www.hannasomatics.com/practitioners

Continuum Movement

Developed by Emilie Conrad (http://continuummovement.com), this is Somatics-style super slow movement without the structure of repetitious movements or deliberately isolating a muscle group. It is neither better nor worse than Somatics, but sometimes, Body has a need to show us how it needs to unwind its tension without imposing a structure.

In Continuum, I allow my body to lead me where the movement wants to take me, which can also lead to epiphany and spontaneous vibrational release of sound that Body wants to make. Practicing Continuum Movement regularly can allow me to make great strides in connecting deeply with Body and embodying my spirit within, via breath and release.

Dreamwalking

Developed by Bee Wolf-Ray (http://earthmatrix.net), dreamwalking is a guided meditation to help the receiver find herself deeply within her Body's consciousness, discovering what characters within the Self come into play and which messages they have for us. A dreamwalking session always begins with a lengthy embodying meditation where the receiver is brought deeply within the locus of the physical body, counter to many guided meditations which have an agenda to move the spirit's consciousness out of the body.

This groundbreaking approach allows for self-connection at levels that can be rarely attained otherwise.

What Is The Physical Body?

Our physical body is not all of us, but hosts the emotional, mental and spiritual bodies. Ideally, if we did not store old pain, we would maintain balance across all our bodies and participate in each realm of ourselves as we are drawn to.

When the physical body presents pain and thereby reveals imbalance, the pain stored is often rooted in old emotional pain. If I participated in every suggestion thus far in this section of the book on a daily basis, I still would not manifest health and balance if I did not do the emotional, mental and spiritual work necessary to manifest overall health within the entire Self. All layers of the being must be healed, and when healing and dealing is applied, old habits are eventually discarded for new, healthier changes which begin to flow in naturally.

If we were to merely focus on healing the symptoms of physical body imbalance alone while ignoring other layers of the self, the body would need constant, repetitive help. Body would not be able to become self-sufficient in any way or clear itself of backlogged pain, make strides and evolve. It therefore becomes crucial to deal with underlying causes for physical issues. This part of Healing and Dealing represents one layer of taking full responsibility for our own healing into wholeness and balance.

* * * * * * * *

Part II

The Emotional Body

This book, beginning primarily with this section, is really only intended for those who feel enough fear, anger or any other emotion in their lives for it to be a problem for them, at least occasionally, where fearful things tend to manifest and are experienced too often as unsafe triggers, aka "reversals of fortune".

The recommendations in this section are not intended for everyone. Some people never seem to get unsafe triggers in their lives, nor are they urged to express emotions for any reason. This can be an indicator that these recommendations of emotional expression (which in the course of the book I will refer to as emotional "movement" or "vibration") are not something these people need to apply. It is also possible that these people have a lot to "move" and just have never opened the door since reaching adulthood. In either case, no one drawn to this book or repelled by it is inferior or superior for their position relative to its content.

However, for someone who has problems with unsafe triggering scenarios, who is experiencing too many reversals of fortune without being able to resolve them, or feels as if they are drowning in or impacted by unresolved emotions rising to the surface, the recommendations for emotional process work delineated in this section and throughout this book can help. With intention and practice, learning to vibrate emotions with smaller triggers can bring safe, or "proactive" triggers into our lives in greater abundance than unsafe, or "reactive" triggers. What is meant by this is, the more you practice the tenets in this book, if you are drawn to, the more you will be able to move feelings in advance of these reversals instead of in response to them. Thus, the process of Healing and Dealing can become less arduous over time, and life's pleasures can be manifested in greater abundance than before.

Be aware that this is a long-term process that requires some dedication and will not completely turn your life around after just a few practices. Lasting internal and external change takes the time it takes depending on how old and deep the blocked emotions are and how strongly denied the emotional body is for each unique person. Yet we have to begin somewhere, and I have found that the more I engage my process, the easier and better life gets overall.

* * * * * * * *

Chapter 7: Emotional Expression and Denial

How often have we heard the phrase "Body, Mind, and Spirit" bandied about? Or how about "the Father, the Son, and the Holy Ghost" to put it a more traditional way? It is practically a cliché that our culture sidesteps or looks past the feminine principle. This principle, Mother energy, is inextricably linked to emotions. Regardless of our gender, the Mother energy within us is our emotional body, containing qualities with soft, purring features like desire, receptivity and intuition. And, let's face it, the emotional side of Mother energy has been thoroughly denied in most of us at some point, even in women.

As consciously growing adults, many of us have begun edging towards acceptance of our emotional reality. We are occasionally starting to notice when we are angry, sad, feeling hurt or scared. Other times, we just know we do not feel good, but we do not know why.

Expression Is the Key

The following quote was taken from a discussion on emotions from a well-known social networking website: "Emotions are not thought about. Emotions are experienced. Emotions are felt. Emotions are sensed. Emotions are integrated into our consciousness through feeling the sensations in our body."

39

I would also like to add to this list a key piece of the puzzle...emotions can be expressed through the body via physical movement, sound or tears. Allowing our triggered emotions to make wordless sound causes an increase in the emotions' vibration that evolves them from their current state of relative stasis, quietude, or outright denial. Depending on the person, this state runs the gamut from utter suppression on the most denied end to noting/feeling/sensing but rarely expressing on the other pole of the denial spectrum.

When the emotions are expressed, they vibrate, and when they vibrate, they evolve, and as they evolve, they release the buried treasure of understanding so that I become consciously aware of what the root cause of the emotion is (often different than the surface trigger that stirred the emotion to life). This is a synergistic experience of spirit, mind, emotions and body where, once enough expression has occurred, healing happens.

Among Our Earliest Messages: Shut Up

Denial is hereditary, passed down through generations. As our society matures, many parents are no longer swatting their children for emotionally expressing sound, as many of our parents and their parents did. Still, the encouragement to deny expression is everywhere. Denial is there in the well-meaning parent joggling a baby to "help her stop fussing", it is there in distracting young children with TV and videos and food rewards if they would just quiet down, it is there in laws and social mores that discourage adults from being outwardly emotional, especially loudly.

A friend of mine, a new mother, could not understand why her five-month-old was constantly whiny and seemingly unhappy for a large part of his days. It did not seem to be a physical discomfort, as she routinely went through the standard solutions of nipple, new diaper, burping, etc., none of which appeared to help him.

I sat down with the baby for a few minutes. He was sitting up on a blanket, fussing away, while Mom walked away for a brief while. As the baby cried and yelled, he held eye contact with me. I let the baby know I accepted his expression.

"Yes, it's hard isn't it," I said gently. "You go right ahead and let me know how hard it really is." His expression amped up slightly. I simply sat and held eye contact as he cried and sounded, clearly surprised that a grownup would encourage him to sound off, largely by staying with him while not attempting to stop or distract him. I held an intent to be with him as long and loud as he wanted to go. I did not try to steer or alter the course his emotions were taking in order to clear themselves. Not long afterward, he quieted, having been allowed to completely finish whatever it was he needed to express. He was witnessed, accompanied and unhindered, and that allowed his emotional body to clear the layer that was up for him rather swiftly and easily.

Two months later I received a call from his mom, who let me know that from that day forward, her baby no longer seemed "colicky" or had long crying jags for no apparent reason. Sometimes acceptance is all the emotional body needs in order to clear itself of old charge. There can be acceptance of others, such as in the story of myself and the baby, only if one has fully enough accepted their own emotions. Otherwise, the "other" will sense the unreleased judgments and lack of acceptance and this won't be effective. We need to focus first on deeply accepting our own internal emotional process before becoming truly effective in helping others accept theirs. Ceasing the "management" of emotions is often what is called for, regardless of the age of the expresser.

Expression, *Then* Understanding

Emotional expression has cycles. It revs up, it peaks, it cycles down, and stasis occurs. Then integration occurs, understandings come in whatever degree they come. Sometime thereafter the next trigger happens, and on and on we go. Our fear of and judgments about expression say that it will get worse, or that particular expression sessions will never end. We fear we will become slaves to our feelings.

Emotional expression needs to come first, seeking mental understandings second. We have traditionally pushed for the other way around. Here's an exchange most of us have heard before:

"Why are you angry?"

"I don't know why I'm angry, I'm just angry!"

"But what's it about?" [subtext: "...so I know it's justified, and therefore I can support its existence"] It is antithetical, hostile, and negating to the emotional body to require justification and explanation for its strength and breadth ahead of allowing its complete cycle of movement and integration.

The attempt to mentally justify whether to express or not has been used against the emotional body. Justifying ahead of expressing has resulted in emotions missing the window of opportunity to release when they are at flashpoint, a window which often can be as small as a second or less. The judgments present here range from labels of insanity to a stern message of "unjustified rage (or any "unjustified" emotion) should not be allowed, since there's no apparent 'good' reason for it", and everything in between.

Emotions are never wrong to exist. When I communicate about how it felt, I am in the land of the subjective, having left the judgmental minefield of the land of the objective. I am on the right track because my feelings are not wrong. They are not objectively accurate via some assessment by an outside person, but they are real to me, and so, they are true for me, and thus, 'never wrong'.

Every emotion is valid. Emotions are natural functions of a healthy body. Their roots may be sourced in past trauma, as a lot of our current emotions are charged to the extent they are due to a backlog of suppressed expression, and therefore may seem unreasonable or unjustifiable in proportion to the trigger. This is also why it is crucial to move in private, as the triggering person is often not the source of the triggered emotion. But even if they are, the charge is more efficiently released in private away from the triggerer. Doing so also helps us to shift from blaming to true transformational expression

The "why's" of our misfired lives are hidden underneath the emotions and often cannot be accessed mentally until the feelings of anger, grief, hurt and fear have had their say. I have found many clear understandings about what is going on with me after I have expressed emotion, but could not find that level of clarity beforehand, no matter how much I tried to get clear before expressing my feelings first.

Suggestions for Safe Expression, Alone or With Others

Some suggestions: Find safe ways to express that do not verbally or physically harm you or others. Hit soft things or yell into down pillows to block your sound if sound safety is an issue. Ask your higher power to fill you with loving light. Create healing circles with your peers and uncover your own denial within that group; this can be a do-it-yourself process with the occasional support of those who do the same thing in their lives. A therapist is not always necessary.

A young boy is continually shushed, yelled at and sometimes punished for expressing anger spontaneously in sound in the house where he lives. One day he breaks his arm in a "freak accident". It is highly likely that this boy, whose avenues for outer expression were continually denied him, unconsciously drew to himself an outlet for his rage the only way it could express – through a violent hurt to the self. Anger turns inward when it is not allowed out, and works against the Self. Denied anger, whether denied by oneself or another, is active energy forced into inactivity, and pressure builds until an outlet is found, even a destructive one.

Tips for Getting To Ignition

Many of us have spent so long bolstering our ability to deny how our emotions would really rather express that there lie hidden many now-subconscious defenses against letting the given emotion on top fully surface. What that means in practical terms is that although we might feel more encouraged to or aligned with allowing our emotions to express than before, we might still have a difficult time getting to the tipping point where these emotions translate into sound or tears. This point is called *ignition*. Other terms used interchangeably here are *activation* or *flashpoint*.

Here are some tips for getting to ignition:

1) When you find yourself triggered, breathe fully, letting the air fill your belly, then bringing the breath upward all the way through the chest cavity, all in one deep inhalation. Let the breath fall out right away, do not hold it and do not push it out. Oftentimes when we are triggered but unconsciously holding tight, we hold our breath or breathe shallowly. I find that opening my breath can open me for ignition.

2) Touch the part of your body you feel is holding the trigger. You can combine this with step 1. Feel in your body, especially over the chakras, where your body is holding the trigger. Put your hand there, just be with yourself there, and bring your inner awareness to this place...feel the quality of energy (swirling, queasy or locked and hard) there and breathe right into it. If doing this does not get you to ignition, imagine a "sleeve" shape opening in the chakra where you feel the pain/tension/energy. Imagine the sleeve continuing from the chakra right to your throat, and invite the energy to rise up and out of your mouth in sound. Invite this energy simply with your unspoken intention and without pushing (emotions do not appreciate being pushed). Allowing even the slightest little river of sound can un-dam the larger pool to which it is connected.

3) Another option to get to flashpoint is to make a "false" sound, a self-conscious noise or sound that is not really the natural expression of the emotion, but rather, sound that is intended to just open the throat chakra. Making a steady "false sound" can connect to organic, real sound that takes on a life of its own until it resolves, which it always does. You will be able to intuitively tell the difference when the organic sound of the emotion takes over.

4) Make yourself a playlist of triggering music, maybe one for rage, one for terror, and one for grief, so you can play the appropriate one for what is on top for

you. Once you have these ready to go, create a ritual. Make a safe inner and outer space for yourself. You can light a candle, say some prayers, set a strong intent to allow your emotional body to take over "control". Call on whatever name for the Divine works for you to join you in this process, and ask for help in getting you to ignition. You can then start the music and assume a comfortable position lying on the floor or sitting up, whichever feels right. Close your eyes and try steps 1 & 2 in combination with this fourth step, and be ready to surrender to your emotional process.

5) If none of this is working, try getting yourself a body-centered psychotherapist just until you can unlock the door to your emotional body and get your emotional backlog in motion. By lying on a table in a body-centered psychotherapy session, and having a practitioner placing their hands on various parts of your body who dialogues with you about how your body feels in those areas, you can be gently and safely assisted to get to some of the deeper feelings stored in your body. Find a practitioner who will allow you the greatest freedom to let your emotional release lead you.

It is not acceptable for a practitioner to attempt to steer your movement. Be aware of the possibility of this happening, and be prepared to see another practitioner if necessary. However, if a practitioner can help you get to the point of release and help you get accustomed to releasing while having the wisdom to back off as soon as you are moving, they are worth their weight in gold. I had the good fortune in my early days of emotional release to live with a student of the art of body-centered psychotherapy who excelled at it, and this was how I had most of my first half-dozen or so significant emotional movements.

When triggered by an external source, I am being presented with a useful and healing opportunity. Many of us have been conditioned to experience triggers as unwelcome. Yet after a few transformational experiences with owning our emotional response and finding the deeper cause or source underneath these emotions, in the end getting great clarity from it all, we can start seeing these events as opportunities. Initial resistance can fall away more quickly than before. Often I hear from proponents of healing and dealing, by the end of a piece of emotional work, the phrase "thanks for the trigger!"

Letting Go Versus Expression

With regards to the New Age philosophy adapted from other disciplines of the past of "letting go" of the feelings, via deep breathing, visualization, noticing and loving them before wishing them or sending them away to the light or down into the earth, etc., know that it is not really possible to let go of parts of the self. If this method could truly work, our world would already show a completely healed and balanced reflection to us.

Feelings are meant to be transitory experiences that spice, highlight and enhance our lives, like a musical soundtrack. When an experience cannot be processed because there are judgments or controls on the natural emotional response to that experience, the experience *and the response* become frozen in time within the self. This frozen place is still within the self, though not as readily accessible, until triggered. Frozen emotional essence is magnetic, and will literally *draw similar experiences into manifestation to the one(s) in which it previously froze* in order to trigger its release.

Emotions cannot be let go of without creating a hole or gap in the self, and even if the letting go is temporarily a success, this emotional essence cannot really go very far. The feelings must be truly released and not just cut off or sent off. When banishing or cutting off emotions happens, parts of us get split off along with the emotions these parts are carrying. These parts of self will need recovery eventually. Releasing the old feelings allows the feelings and the parts of self holding them to evolve without pushing any part of ourselves away.

Release in this case means emotional expression in sound and body movement, with minimal control on how the sounds express. The meaning of the word release in this context is not "letting go" as in "sending away"; in this context release is akin to noticing there is a coiled spring in your hand, and then loosening the hand so the spring can stretch and extend to its real, uncontrolled length.

It is much easier and healthier to process the feelings as they occur than to try to recover old, frozen, darkened, repressed emotional reactions that have been pushed out of the self for months, years, or decades. Unfortunately, we have all been taught how or commanded to perform attempts at casting out or repressing these emotions. As children many of us attempted to comply with such teachings or commands as a survival technique (to please our parents, keep them giving us love and support if we comply with them, prevent punishments, etc.) and we have attained varying degrees of mastery at it, depending upon whether our intrinsic nature as an individual leans more to the electric side of Self (i.e. more generally masculine) or the magnetic (more generally feminine).

Emotional Projection

Projection is a hallmark of our misunderstanding about and inexperience with dealing with long-held powerful emotions. Resolving emotions fully is what permits me to take personal responsibility for them in any kind of real, gut-level way. It is very easy to project an unfelt, unacknowledged emotion. With experience it becomes easier to know even in advance of expressing the charge of the emotion that it is really mine.

People in leadership positions are projected upon all the time as the mommy/daddy who never gave enough or in the right way. The projections come from people carrying hurt feelings of victimization, originally at the hands of their parents. These victimized-feeling people are carrying very old, enraged and hurt feelings deep in their background, feelings related to what they did not get as children. They acquired these old feelings originally in justifiable ways, but the ones who become the projection screens in the now are their triggers, new targets of the same old held blame carried forward. The triggered people do not even realize that they are projecting past, still-held trauma onto the leader of the moment. Most of them do not even realize they are triggered. In this they are simply acting out the emotions instead of feeling and expressing them appropriately.

These people attract situations to match/trigger their unresolved feelings, trying in vain to resolve them by acting out the blame and trying to pin it on anyone who even remotely resembles the original ones they are mad at, hoping at last that some responsibility will be taken by "them". It is an attempt at getting rid of the harsh, old, painful feelings.

This approach never works. They draw scenario after triggering scenario, because the blame never really goes anywhere. This cycle repeats until the emotions are responsibly dealt with at their root, when they are really, effectively released and not just acted out further. Without dealing with the root emotional causes, only a vanishingly small percentage of these people ever seem to be able to resolve these original feelings in any kind of effective way. Healing and dealing, as outlined in this book, raises the chances considerably of breaking through into greater levels of emotional resolution than we had dreamed possible.

Resolving hurt feelings of victimization largely involves expressing all of the emotions involved: the deep, bitter, hurt tears, the rages at mistreatment, and the fear of further victimization any new authority figures bring up for these people. Forgiveness for judging ourselves, others and our environment will flow naturally at some point when enough emotion is expressed. Eventually a root-level understanding will be gleaned where victim and perpetrator are recognized as two sides of the same person.

From Misunderstanding to Responsibility

We all have had to wrestle with myriad misunderstandings about emotions and their true nature, and most of us are just beginning to learn how to accept our emotionality fully. We had poor teachers and role models in our elders, because they did not have any helpful emotional role models either. The pattern extends all the way back up the ancestral tree. Ours is the first generation to be gifted with an awareness of what works to clear emotions at their roots and evolve them, thus clearing our whole being, layer by layer.

As we grow and evolve our emotional centers and clear out the layers of denial we have accrued for countless lifetimes, we start to realize at an intuitive level that we are little microcosms of the One. Therefore, when we have feelings, we can be sure they say something about us when, over time and deeds, we get better at listening and "speaking her language" (the feminine emotional aspect of ourselves). We begin to hear more fully from our emotional intelligence, taking on faith that ultimately, everything is about us, even if we cannot always quite see how.

As we grow, our faith deepens that we will glean a true understanding if we nurture our intent to hear such truth, asking and desiring deeply to KNOW, once and for all, what our involvement and responsibility is in a given situation. The more we redeem our emotions from their state of denial, the easier this inquiry/discovery process becomes.

Many Roads

If you try a path of emotional expression for a good long time and find that it does not feel right for you, or you find yourself organically pulling away from it while realizing that doing so does not feel the same as avoidance, perhaps this healing modality is not right for you at this time. Nobody knows the true path for another. You can also ask your Higher Power, Spirit, Deeper Self, or whatever term for the Divine suits you to give you guidance in a form you can hear on how to deal with your feelings. This could be a "sign", a dream, an inner voice or some other way that is just right for you. Remember to watch and listen for an "answer", something you can recognize as help.

If after all this you are convinced that the emotions are not yours, perhaps they are not. You could then ask Spirit to remove any fear that is not your own and put it where it belongs. If nothing changes, then one possibility is that the fear is yours, and it will require you to release its backed-up charge, a little at a time, layer by layer, from having been denied for so long, so it can be transmuted into love and trust. All of this can be accomplished by expressing emotionally in sound and tears when you are triggered. The process doesn't have to be more complicated than that.

Another possibility is that the owner of these emotions has not redeemed them and the emotions have split off him or her onto you. This is the phenomenon known as essence fragmentation. These feelings are not your responsibility. When the ultimate owner's experiences trigger them to undertake the emotional work that touches the particular emotional energy you are storing, you may have the experience of having something simply lifted off of you and feeling lighter without having done anything to cause it. Or, as another example, you may have a physical accident in order to jar the stuck energy loose, after recovery from which you feel "changed in some way". In either scenario if you then find you are not afraid of the same things as before the change, it is a good bet that those feelings went to their right place and were able to evolve.

If none of the above works, you could try a therapy group that encourages emotionality. You can go into it with an intention of resolving issues you normally project onto others, with a curiosity to discover what your strong feelings about others say about you. Shop around for a group that feels right to you; you are worth the effort. If you have strong intent to change your emotional patterns then you are very likely to find the help you need.

Men Need To Heal and Deal

Why do we teach boys not to cry? Because men have been seen, and still are in many people's minds, as society's strength, and holding back emotions is equated with strength, stoicism=strength, etc. These perceptions need to go the way of the dinosaur.

Repressed emotions are killing men, and in turn traumatize society in general when the repressed emotions act out in various ways. Express emotions safely and in private safe space, and all will improve.

Another problem with men and emotions is the outdated concept of "rugged individualism", a.k.a. "I don't need no help from nobody". Many boys were conditioned to believe this by their fathers' modeling and society at large. I have struggled with this one too, and am getting better asking for help nowadays when I need it, but my programming taught the opposite.

The stress of chronically holding back emotions and letting stress pile up because we men feel we have to do it all ourselves is a 1-2 punch that regularly sends us down.

There is also a big healing "bonus" somewhere in here, when a man can find a trusted other(s) who they can cry or express with and to. This is gold when we can find such people to help witness us if we want or need that.

Emotions Can Grow Up Too

It is said that certain emotions acting out in people make them look childish. That is not a bad description. These feelings are *not* grown up. They are indeed unevolved when they act out. When the person acting out makes somebody else the problem, they are revealing that they have yet to grow up emotionally in that particular area.

Over time, expressing emotions in sound and body movement curbs so-called childish behavior, because expressing these emotions instead of acting them out, and receiving resultant understandings about what they are really about helps them to "grow up" or catch up with the rest of the self.

I grew up hearing the phrase, "The less you do, the less you want to do". A version of this old adage is apropos here, although finding emotions is not at all about "doing" or pressuring one's self to work harder. Still, the tendency is the less you are in touch with your emotions, the less you want to be. It takes a conscious willingness and intentional effort to go there. To really evolve the emotions trapped in the past, one has to really *want* to find them in order to evolve. Like anything else, this gets easier with practice.

Chapter 8: Sound and Safety

Private or safe space is crucial for effective emotional expression. People on the path of emotional expression use sound blockage so as not to viscerally blow away the eardrums of people who might be sitting within close range. They also use blockage so that if there is someone within earshot who might be tempted to report you to the authorities for making loud or "strange" sound, you will not be heard. Soft, deeply-squishy pillows are ideal sound blockage. Pressing the pillow closely around the face and coming up for air when necessary is simple and effective. Ideally, people would normally carry towels around with them, in case they need to move feelings.

Clearly towels are more convenient than pillows away from home, though they block less sound. They do block enough sound, however, to lessen the effect of your expression on people nearby. If, for example, you needed to express sound in a wooded area that was relatively close to civilization, a towel or even a handkerchief would be enough to block the sound outside a radius of 50-75 yards.

Pillows would not be necessary in cases where one was not sitting around the house with others nearby, because pillows in particular are meant to make it so someone in the next room or upstairs or whatever would not even be able to *know* you were expressing. Sometimes the emotional body is terrified of being found out to be making loud or weird sounds and be penalized or shamed in some way by someone else feeling a need to "check out the disturbance." Knowing the people within earshot and whether they are likely to actively participate in shutting you down is essential. Helping the emotional body feel safe to express by blocking your sound is a very important step in the emotional healing process.

Sometimes I find that sound does NOT want to be blocked or controlled in its expression, in terms of volume, style, or dynamics. Finding sound-safe space where nobody's ears will be impinged upon and nobody is likely to hear you or care to stop you if they did hear you is a gift, when available. Many emotional expressers have limited safe space availability, so achieving safe space, sometimes creatively, is important too. Cars, forests, ducking under the water, and rooms in houses when nobody is home or the music is turned up loud are gold for safe space.

The Importance of Safe Release Space

I do not release in public, and I do not recommend it be tried unless holding back until you get to a private sound-secure space feels impossible. The emotional body usually desires and requires more safety than that. Occasionally, with a group I feel safe with, I might take a chance and express in their presence, and then only in very special and extreme circumstances, as I did once outside a sweat lodge (a spiritually-oriented space) Even then, I keep a protective eye out with part of me. Safety is important with emotional expression. Babies can "get away" with expressing in public and sometimes older children, but not adults, not as our culture stands now.

There is a movement afoot nearly everywhere in today's version of reality that has, as its ultimate agenda, to stamp out spontaneous emotional sound entirely so "peace and quiet" will reign and no pesky emotions ever need to be dealt with or experienced again either from within or from without. This acts out as repression of anyone trying to express big in others' presence or earshot, to the point of incarceration and hospitalization, the latter of which of course most often includes enforced drugging with sedatives and heavy-duty antidepressants. Forms of lobotomy are still practiced for adults expressing in sound. This is no exaggeration; notice the powers that be increasing repression of civil rights, or the controlling of free will.

In the face of such intimidating opposition from certain quarters "out there", safety in the form of private, sound-secure space for emotional expression is needful in today's world. In an ideal world, everyone would have some level of acceptance for emotional expression, at least a little bit, and so moving into towels, hankies or pillows would reveal that "yeah that person is expressing some feelings over there" but it would not be so loud as to overwhelm the people nearby. In that kind of world an adult expressing emotion would not be considered any bigger deal than a baby crying or yelling.

"Free" Will?

Will is not free on this planet, not yet, not by a long shot. Will means many things, and there are many sub-layers. Among many other aspects, the will is another name for the emotional body. Free will includes the power of expression, the power to "do as thou wilt, with intent to harm none". Freedom of will includes feeling desire and taking action to satisfy that desire, the freedom to respond to intention and inspiration. Freedom of will to *not* respond because there is no organic desire is also part of free will. The human will is the freedom of movement and action "just because I feel like it in *this* moment". A free will in balance does not harm or overpower others, or infringe on others' freedoms without a win-win being found. We have precious little of that kind of freedom around us, so far, if we really look closely.

Instead, we have structures of intimidation like police and jail and hospitals and courtrooms and churches and overpowering parents that control and repress the movement of free will, emotional expression, civil rights. This is why safe, relatively quiet and private space for expression is going to be needful until Earth shifts and we regain our collective empowerment, leaving no more space for any unloving agenda of oppression and control. At that point, guilt goes away for good, and balance and common understanding of what is supportive of life appears everywhere that unlovingness and guilt have been.

Earth Changes and Emotional Expression

It will not likely be safe for mass movement in public until some major manifestation of what has come to be called "Earth Changes" by some are in full swing, and expression becomes more normalized as a result. Public emotional expression would be safer if Earth Changes were in our faces because most people would not be able to hold back anymore with all the concomitant catastrophe, or whatever is going to end up as "the next world" starts coming into place. In other words, if most of us were doing it because we were so triggered we could not hold back, expression would become more normalized.

However, in the face of Earth Changes – potentially catastrophic changes to our immediate as well as our global environment - how I *hold* my emotional body means everything in terms of how its expression would manifest under such extremes of pressure. If I love and actively embrace my will and her feelings, granting them enough acceptance for and understanding of the pain they have had to repress and hold back over the eons, then I will have weaker judgments against what I end up expressing in the face of extreme triggering that such Earth Changes may bring. My journey through the gauntlet of personal pain as society "phoenixes" itself through a major death and rebirth cycle will be that much smoother because I am ready and able to walk the fire. I would be ready and able to take it to the next level, bringing all of myself to bear and not leaving anything behind, including my previously denied emotions.

On the other hand, the less I have practiced organic emotional expression, the less aware I am of what is going on in my emotional denials. When we chronically deny, our emotional suppleness is lacking, and we are rigid and still. It also follows that in such a state we have very strong judgments against allowing emotional expression. The more judgments we inherently hold on our wills the more they will act, when pressured, to "satisfy" or match the judgments they have been burdened with by our minds and input from similar points of view outside us

For example, let's say I was a person who judged emotional expression as childish and immature. I then faced a situation where I was triggered so heavily as to overcome my resistance to expressing emotionally. My expression may well act out in childish and immature ways. I may face those judgments from the people around me, or be judging myself all the way along for "how I am behaving." Such a scenario does not reflect acceptance of my emotions under duress, and thus the emotions cannot express appropriately and heal in the face of such weight of judgment. The emotional body, in short, does not open in the face of lack of acceptance for its natural expression. Similarly, my emotions do not act openly and cleanly if they break loose despite strong resistance and clampdown.

However, if I am ready for such intense triggering that Earth Changes might bring, because I have been practicing free expression of my emotions in safe and appropriate ways, I can give myself the greatest chance of using crisis as a means to take a quantum leap in my personal evolution. I will be able to use crisis as a springboard, a steppingstone, and perhaps not encounter major reversal, or at least, as major as it would have been otherwise. Acceptance, practice and release of beliefs about what emotional expression is will carry me a long way towards being able to emotionally and physically survive potential catastrophe.

Ideally, we are collectively moving enough old, denied emotions proactively, so as to experience smaller, less impactful triggers than heavy Earth Changes to get us off the emotional dime. I continue to envision and pray for a more graceful transition to whatever the new world is going to look like. Together, however, we really have to be there, enough of us have to be doing this work deeply to ameliorate a harsh reflection in order to transmute and heal our society.

Chapter 9: The Backlog of Emotional Charge

Genevieve hurls insults at her partner when he says she should know better than to trust her doctor to give her the right advice for her injured foot. She leaves the room crying. Later, she tells a girlfriend that she overreacted.

People often believe that if their emotional response is out of proportion to the trigger at hand, they have "overreacted". Emotions when triggered are too often misunderstood as overreactions. It is used as a categorical label to describe a reaction misunderstood because it is not logically proportionate to the "weight" of the surface trigger. Yet children, our emotional teachers, sometimes cry voluminously at the slightest injury, taking advantage of every opportunity to offload accumulated emotional charge.

Instead of labeling Genevieve's true response an overreaction, we could say she reacted exactly in proportion to the backlog of held emotions accrued across her entire lifetime (some would say, lifetimes) in the area of her will in which she was triggered. The word "overreact" connotes that she was out of line for having the response she did. The concept of overreaction also reveals a widely held judgment that one's emotional reaction should be controlled to match, but not exceed, the exact level of response stirred by the trigger at hand – input in, input out, the modus operandi of a machine or computer. The emotional body does not operate under the same rules of logic as a robot, or even the mental body; yet, when considering all that has been emotionally denied in our existential history, the emotional body functions in a perfectly logical manner.

Eliminate The Kneejerk Reaction?

Attempted non-reaction is not healing and dealing either. My friend Carmen wrote to me relating her attempts to suppress her initial angry response in a potential "road rage" scenario: "What I hope is happening when I 'refuse" to feel or ventilate road rage is eliminating the knee jerk reaction. I think we are somewhat programmed to feel *entitled* to be angry when we perceive an insult."

Yes, this is an example of that old righteous indignation thing, where we are "justifiably" enraged. "How dare they do that to me!" This comes from believing we have no responsibility for our experiences. This is another way we are programmed, whereby "everything that happens to us is random," or we adopt a superior stance: "I would NEVER do that". We feel entitled to strike back because of our cultural revenge imprint; miniature pitchfork devils whisper in our ears that "the score must be evened".

Carmen continues, "It does not feel like I'm burying it, it feels like I'm refusing to rise to the bait."

Emotional responses are immediate and natural. If your reaction is kneejerk or seemingly out of proportion to the trigger, and you prefer a different response, then how to address that first reaction? Refusing to "rise to the bait" means refusing to acknowledge the reaction, therefore denying that you are having the reaction by enforcing calm as a secondary response. Emotional re-action is a defense mechanism that cannot be bypassed if we want to get to the deeper, natural emotionally triggered response underneath the reaction.

The debate here is whether that first reaction is real. Instead of substituting a second response, one could address healing that initial, 'kneejerk' response by healing over time so that one no longer has the same over-the-top response to the same stimuli, ad infinitum. People on an emotional healing path see this process as an opportunity to unwind some compressed, precious emotional energy that becomes life-giving when decompressed and expressed fully.

Thar Be Treasure Below!

If upon hearing such rationale you think "what a masochist!" know that underneath all that pain - and it IS finite, if massive - lies denied joy. This is real, endless joy, not the kind of momentary joy that is an interlude in a seemingly never-ending litany and dull reality of pain, suppression, duty and gray colorless days of routine existence. Treasure indeed exists beneath all the harsh feelings.

Underneath our so-called "negative" emotional backlog of anger, fear, and grief that we so often do not even know is there until it gets triggered, lies the gold -- spontaneity, laughter, childlike earnestness and more. It seems to be the nature of the beast that when we deny the hard feelings, the ones we would like to experience go away as well, to one degree or another. The spontaneous and joyful gifts of childhood are the casualties of inner and outer repression.

With patience, perseverance and willingness to express everything we feel in the form of sound, tears and/or body movement as a top priority, we will, over time and shovelful by shovelful dig down to this storehouse of birthrights.

We can have this treasure but we will not have it in never- ending supply until the unevolved emotional backlog is healed. To get there many of us need to feel and express our old feelings first. You will know if the emotional healing path is right for you if this book has a resonance for you and you try out the suggestions within and notice positive results.

Healthy open expression of anger and emotions such as grief, hurt and fear seems farfetched because we live in a culture of denial, where holding them in is seen as natural. When something has been practiced for millennia, it seems that must be the right way. I disagree that it is the right way; holding feelings back as a matter of course does not lead to healing. As Sinead O'Connor once sang, "Life's backwards, life's backwards/People, turn around".

How I Broke The Ice, And What Happened Next

An acquaintance in her early 20s wrote to me during a discussion about expressing vulnerable emotions. She said that the thought of showing her innermost and tender feelings and therefore becoming vulnerable felt just unbearable. She said she felt very terrified of her emotions.

I let her know that this was exactly how I felt at her age. It was unquestionable to me then that if I dared cry even a little about anything in any kind of "allowing" way (other than when a tear glistened my eye against all manner of attempt at holding back) I would be lost forever. The dragon in the closet was a leviathan, the hideous devil himself, I was certain of it! Never give an inch or I will be lost forever! Never EVER let down my guard! All subconscious dictates of course.

This approach to my denied emotions melted juhhhhhhhhhst enough around my Saturn Return (age 28-30 for everyone) for me to surprise myself with a two hour crying jag on a healing table while someone ran energy into my body a la Reiki while asking me questions about my past, my parents, etc. In responding, I cracked the door, my emotions spilled out, and my expression of them had a natural ending. At the two hour mark my healing facilitator ran out of steam and left me alone to integrate my experience. I'd started meditating around that time in my life, and so had a glimpse of spiritual energy. I trusted by then that there was some kind of Loving Light presence beyond me, greater than me, that could support me through this storm.

When I finally got up, I remember crawling around on the floor, still crying a little bit, muttering THANK YOU THANK YOU THANK YOU to nobody in particular, or maybe to myself for daring to let the pressure out of the cooker. I then sobbed over and over, I NEED MORE OF THIS, I NEED MORE OF THIS!!! I remember it so clearly, both the experience and the feeling of relief and gratitude afterward. Standing on this side of the denial door I could see for the first time that it was way harder to expend the minute-to-minute effort it took to hold back the flood than to let some of it out. And I learned, first hand (nobody could have told me in a way I could have believed, prior) that I could survive the experience, that there was a natural endpoint. What a concept! Nearly thirty years and hundreds and hundreds of similar and sometimes even greater releases later, I have learned that I can survive every single emotional release experience. I learned that there is always an organic endpoint to what's ready to release and express, what's on top, no matter how big or all-encompassing it feels during the release.

After that initial experience, I had about half a dozen more like it on my practitioner's table, exploring not just existential grief but huge rage in wordless screaming sounds. She and I were becoming romantically involved, and so she stepped aside as my "healer" at that point (really, I was healing myself, she was helping out). After that, I took control of my own process. I could feel so thoroughly that it was my path to move as much of this pure emotion as I could. I used to light a candle, all alone at home, say a few prayers for myself, make sure the kleenex box was nearby, turn the lights out and then spin the most triggering music I had in my collection, the kind I always had to hold back sooooooo intensively when I heard before. I decided that without a doubt even in those early days that not only could I survive the experiences, but that I would be better off for allowing them.

Slowly but surely, I got "better". I became less filled to the brim with unexplored tears, fears, rages and hurts. My ability to deny my experiences and my triggers weakened, by my own choice to quit denying how I really felt. I became slowly but surely more emotionally confident. I got sick less. I got injured less. I had fewer "accidents". I had gradually fewer reversals in my life. My energy was stronger, better. My body started healing and loosening up. My walk changed; my face changed (not just with age!). I started feeling less guilty and more confident. I found that my patterns actually changed; I wasn't always so predictable to myself or others in how I would react to certain things. In fact, my reactions to certain stimuli shifted - things that would trigger me so badly before stopped doing so the more I allowed myself to have my organic emotional response to them.

Deeply emotional people have well developed denial muscles. They either have to, or they learn to swim in the dark water. I'm a really strong swimmer now. My "muscles" were all bulky and stony. Once I learned how to release my emotions in sound and tears, they got more and more streamlined and supple.

from A to U

sometimes feelings
can't find the right words
& sometimes there are
so many feelings that
they are better not spoken
they are better if sung...
& words are not essential
the heart has its
own wailing songs...
that's why vowels exist...

© Robert J. Dagostino

Chapter 10: Whose Emotions Are These Anyway?

How do you know when the emotions you feel are yours or another's? You cannot necessarily know until after they express, when greater understanding becomes available. Whether yours or theirs, what is happening for you in the moment is a "real" expression. In most cases, you still have to vibrate, via non-verbal emotional expression, the anger, fear or grief out of you, whether the emotion is yours or not. Occasionally you can notice that it is another's emotions that you feel when you take physical distance from these others and suddenly you do not feel these feelings as intensely.

Sometimes an empathic person holds the emotions of another: someone else in the room, maybe a friend, or perhaps a partner. Often, a woman is holding the emotions of her man. Generally speaking, and with exceptions, this is because a woman's energy field tends to be more magnetic in nature, whereas a man's tends to be electric. Electric energy moves quickly, gives of itself and does not hold on to much for long, whereas magnetic energy moves more slowly, receives, attracts and holds on.

Practical Assumption: If I Feel It, It Is Mine

The initial stage to transforming the effect of any old emotion within the self is acknowledging the emotion is yours. We can easily become confused and say the trigger of the emotion is the owner of the emotion, or that we would never be feeling this emotion if it were not for them triggering it. On this tack we then want to change their behavior so our fear or anger can go back to the quiet slumber of denial that it was in before being awakened.

If you are feeling afraid, for instance, assume the fear is yours. If you are feeling angry, assume the anger is yours. Once release happens and true understanding comes in, you will know more deeply if you were returning another's emotions to them by vibrating them off of yourself or if the emotions were yours all along. When awareness flows in to show you the roots of your original response to the trigger and why you denied the emotions in the first place, you know the emotions were yours.

Fear of Rage

I went through a long period in my early years of emotional healing being terrified of rage. I quickly learned I was frightened of my own unmoved (unexpressed) rage. I had to experience enough movement of pure, unfettered rage expression in raw sound to be able to make friends with the vibration of deep anger. This helped me stop feeling victimized when another person in the room was angry. The more I owned my own unprocessed anger, the more I stopped feeling afraid of someone else's rage and of "taking it on".

True Rage Release

Confusion and lack of understanding often accompany rage expression at first. Understandings about whose rage it was and what it was about can seep in days and even weeks later. I sometimes do not feel better immediately after a rage release. The process of releasing rage may not feel good even when my expression is "clean", i.e., in my own space and not blaming someone else in words.

Nevertheless, I have seen over time that as a result of letting anger express in sound that I now have less anger at things and people than I used to. I have received understandings after moving rage that I never had before. These understandings often come in to awareness days later or hours later, not always right away. I usually just feel "bad" for a little while, not "relieved" in the same ways I feel after a good cry or a good fear movement. Conversely, many experienced emotional expressers find anger release wholly satisfying. Your mileage may vary. In either case, there is a softening in the self from transforming the hard rock of held rage via its expression in sound and body movement. That alone makes it worth the effort.

Verbal Versus Primal

There is a difference if I "move" rage in words versus in sound, or jumping up and down and allowing myself a "tantrum", or beating pillows. I have gone out in the woods and used deadfall like a club to smash over larger dead logs. If I just mutter, tell an angry story, write an angry email, sing an angry song or yell blaming words and never get to the primordial sound underneath, I am merely riding the surface. Anyone can dump a bunch of words and just wait for the inevitable subsiding; for that you do not need healing intent. Millions of people do it every day. That method of expressing anger does not heal or evolve the emotion. There may be some temporary feelings of satisfaction but the core of the anger is still there, un-transformed.

It takes more to get at the roots than just words. Words and blaming words are useful, and they can often lead to what I call flashpoint. But in my own process it is important to me to seek a point where I can "drop out" of words, find the flashpoint and move into the full conflagration of primordial, roaring rage. Shift will come after that.

Blaming is saying, in so many words "you are wrong for treating me that way, you are bad, you should have done it another way". On the other hand, noticing and taking responsibility is the act of acknowledging "I did those things", end of story. Saying "I did those things" is different than an assignment of fault or culpability, or a judgment that the emotions or actions involved were good, bad, should not have been done, etc. When we take responsibility for our emotions by acknowledging this responsibility to ourselves or to another, healing begins in earnest and sometimes interpersonal miracles can occur. This taking of responsibility is also known as owning our emotions.

Rage in blaming words, spoken or typed, is a phase in the process of fully owning and expressing the root emotion of anger. It is a step along the way, comprising the final vestiges of resistance to truly and deeply *feeling* the emotion. I am still pushing anger away from me when I blame something or someone. Paradoxically, the phase of wrong-making blame isn't a mistake, and in most cases can't be skipped over without repercussions.

In fully embracing my healing intent in the moment, I allow my rage to make sound. I allow rage to have its deeper, non-verbal say, which in turn helps me rebuild inner empowerment and clarity to both understand and deal more efficiently with the situation at hand.

Cycling

There exists also the pattern of always resorting to anger to mask deeper feelings. That kind of a pattern is called cycling – an emotional habit or grooved response to shunt the awareness away from the more vulnerable feelings underneath. Conversely, cycling in grief or fear can also take place, avoiding feelings of rage. Feeling for what is below the topmost emotion is important if you are expressing repeatedly and seem to not be getting anywhere. We will see in Part III that the judgments we hold against particular emotions play a role in avoiding what is traditionally harder for us to feel or express. Once these judgments are released it can be an easier road to access the avoided emotion if strong intent exists to do so.

What happens with cycling is that there is a subconscious *conversion* from the emotion that has organically arisen into an emotion that is habitually easier to feel. For example, someone who often feels angry will convert grief or terror immediately into anger without knowing it. Even if this person releases and expresses this anger safely every single day, they will not get very far, because they are bypassing or "jumping the gap" between the initial grief or fear response and only noticing anger. Conversely, as I said above, converting in the opposite direction can be just as habitual for certain people, i.e. converting organic feelings of anger to grief, or cycling in hurt or fear.

Chapter 11: Fear of Fear Itself

A friend wondered what feeling her fear was supposed to do for her. She said that whenever fearful pictures arose in her mind, which was often, she suppressed the feelings that came with the pictures.

Acknowledging, accepting, feeling and expressing fear in wordless sound or body movement is often extremely uncomfortable, especially at first. Expressing fear safely and with as much acceptance as you can give it actually relieves the pressured feeling inside that any growing, internalized fear bubbling to the surface gives us. That is what expressing the fear can do for you.

Most people do not even recognize that emotions are a part of the self, and a part that needs healing because of routine, lifetimes-long denial patterns. We cannot successfully cut off parts of ourselves, but that is what we are attempting when we suppress. Emotions are a part of ourselves, and fear only feels bad because we have denied it for so long. Anything that gets routinely denied feels dark, monstrous, alien, and scary. Fear does not feel nearly as bad to me as it used to because I do not deny it nearly as much as I used to.

The Universal Judgment on Fear

Before you feel it, the fear feels like a dragon in the closet; as you go into it and come out the other side, the dragon shrinks away, perhaps to a salamander.

Feeling and expressing fear, or any emotion, in a given area or issue may take several or many passes to get through all the "layers", like peeling an onion. How fast anyone can release fear of something or someone depends on how deep that issue goes and how deep the movement of the fear goes each time you are triggered into it.

The judgment that comes up for nearly everybody who considers expressing fear for the first time or first few times is, "If I dare feel or express this fear, what I am afraid of will manifest". My experience is that the opposite occurs – if I dare to release the fear by allowing its expression it does not need to draw a reflection of itself into manifestation in order to trigger it.

The denial of how afraid we really feel while focusing on mental pictures attracts what we fear. Often if I can release the fear ahead of any fear-inducing event, the event either does not happen or manifests much more benignly than I had originally feared. In this context, "nothing to fear but the denial of fear itself" would be an accurate coining of the old maxim. American president Franklin Delano Roosevelt, the author of the famous quote "There is nothing to fear but fear itself" was not into healing and dealing!

Fear "or" Love

"So what're ya gonna choose, fear or love?" -- the ultimate rhetorical question, posed by smugly smiling gurus of all ilks down through history. There is no possible answer, because the two forces are not oppositional. They are parts of the same whole. Fear is felt by the body in a millisecond. Your choice is to feel it or deny it. It is already there and it is quicker than you are.

Fear is embedded in us from the start, and when the sleeping giant of fear is stirred by an inner or outer event, the real choice around what to do with it is love it (by acknowledging, accepting and expressing how it really feels) or fear it (denying it--pushing it away by mentally lifting out of it with affirmations or a strong intent to avoid, get rid of or "overcome it"). Thus, the choice becomes not one between fear or love, but between acceptance or denial.

Handling Fear in a New Way

Fear is not the problem. It is simply another emotion to be felt, like grief or anger. Fear of fear is the problem. Fear of fear is rooted in judgment and hatred for how it feels to be afraid. This is not wrong; to notice what is in the way of feeling and expressing is actually quite important. If you hate your fear, that is the starting place. Hate it. Go ahead and despise it for making you feel victimized and powerless, but let the hatred blow up big and in sound. Judge your fear, rage at it, spew out loud how much you hate it. Stomp around, imagine putting your fear in a chair and whap the life out of it with pillows or a plastic bat. Doing so can be a bridge to acceptance of fear's reality. Eventually, releasing those judgments about fear is going to be important – more on this in Part III ("The Mental Body").

The intent here needs to be to get to the point of breakthrough regarding your fear. To simply hate on and act out on one's fear as in the previous examples given of hating it or whapping the life out of it with a bat will only work to heal anything if the intent to get to the lost sound expression is fully present, and ideally, arrived at. In a therapy session, I was invited to do just that – when I said my fear was "giving me problems" my therapist had me imagine putting my fear in a chair and letting it know how much I didn't like it, handing me a tennis racket to "kill it". I realize now that he was trying to help me get to flashpoint around it. Instead, with racket raised, I crumpled to the floor in sudden compassion for my fear, and experienced my first fear expression in sound, my face contorting in a way that had never happened to me before. After that, I could express my fear in sound, and it was no longer a "problem" in my life, but simply another emotion to be processed when a new layer was triggered.

The way to truly transform "crunchy" emotions like fear, rage, or hurt is to let the emotions vibrate by allowing the sound to come up from the place in our bodies where we feel the emotion, into our throats and out our mouths as sounds; weird sounds, soft or loud sounds, tears. This is the deepest, most thorough way to organically transform an emotion at its root. We have all tried cutting emotions off as a way to "get rid of them", separating ourselves from the feelings in various ways, but that kind of denial catches up with us sooner or later.

If the sounds you are able to let out are quiet, that's alright. Subtle or soft sounds can feel and be powerful. Soft or small sounds are all that can be allowed sometimes. With time and practice, a stream of sound reflecting the power of the held fear will emerge at times. Sound may go from quiet to loud to quiet, there is no predicting or "right way" for this process to occur.

With unconditional acceptance of the style and volume of your sound, the emotion will have space to be purely itself, exactly how it is ready to come out. Be aware of not forcing anything sound-wise. Allow the sounds to be natural, with the most sensitive presence you can give them, as though your feelings were a friend in distress. Forcing sound can block emotion and create a false mask hiding the true expression of the emotion.

That said, making self-conscious sounds in order to connect with the subconscious sounds silenced within can be an excellent bridge into your organic sound expression and letting it take over.

Fear -> Love -> Trust

I propose the following definition of fear: A deep, non-mental mistrust that something which is perceived to have power over us might hurt us in some way, or an indefinable mistrust of ourselves or another. Mistrust is the keyword. Fear, or any emotion that we have labeled negative can be born *into* love via accepting its presence and allowing its expression. New understandings will fill us when we are done expressing, understandings about why we felt the way we did. Fear or mistrust, once within love, becomes trust.

A big part of our problem with emotional expression is that we have been taught from birth to deny the fullness of our emotional expression. Here we approach the roots of denial. Emotions, if completely accepted for what they are, express themselves in sound.

A baby in its first year of life is a ball of sound. Slowly but surely, inner and outer forces conspire to contain the level, breadth, and freedom of expression until we reach adulthood, when we rarely or never express emotionally in sound. We feel it sometimes rise up from the inner depths still, but we routinely push down the inclination to make sound, which then rises against this resistance anyway, once we have magnetized a particular life experience big enough to trigger it (funny how that works!). Without self-acceptance, that expression looks as twisted and feels as yucky to ourselves and others as we have judged it to be.

"So how will you approach your fear, with fear or with love?"

The Faces of Fear

Worry is a more sublimated form of fear. Worry is the tip of the iceberg of a terror held in the subconscious parts of our being. The continuum looks like this: Worry->anxiety->fear->terror. They are all forms of the same emotion, depending on how much of it is consciously felt in a given area. Fear is an emotion, but is not universally understood, recognized or acknowledged as an emotion, like anger or grief is.

Worry can also be sourced in the mental body. "What if" thoughts sometimes spin round and round inside our minds like hamsters on a wheel. "Dropping beneath" the worry thoughts by stopping what I am doing and feeling inside myself deeply to try to find and express the pocket of deeper emotion signaled by the worry can prove fruitful. Feeling where in my body the fear resides and placing a hand there often helps. Then I can "breathe into" that part of my body, breathe into the fear, welcoming it to tell its story, which can often help me to feel safe enough there to allow expression of what is REALLY bothering me, much more deeply than surface worry thoughts of the moment.

Ways to Release Fear

Many of us have become willing to notice, acknowledge and feel fear in our bodies, seeking to find root cause, but have not fully found evolution in the fear responses we normally have to the same repeated stimuli. This is because a key piece – the expression of the emotion of fear - is not being allowed or is not acknowledged as the key piece.

Most of us misunderstand what expressing emotion really is. We sometimes believe expressing emotion equates to reacting, blaming the other or the situation, battling. These are emotional masks, and source in reactive parts of our brain. We can "cycle" in these reactive places and never drop further down into deeper places and emotions, the ones we really need to feel instead of escaping by blaming the reflection.

Blaming is sometimes necessary as a starting place, a way station on the journey to self-responsibility and true healing. Blaming is also like a cue to notice there are even deeper currents. Blame shows us, eventually, that we have to get vulnerable with ourselves, because eventually, responsibility for our feelings source in us. It's up to us to find, own and express from all the layers in which they exist. This understanding is crucial, because there will be no real healing, no external shift and personal evolution until we access the deeper feeling currents underneath the reaction.

Some of us believe expressing emotion is talking about the feelings. Talking about my fear can be a steppingstone on my way to expressing it, but it is not the expression of the emotion itself. Talking is a mental activity, trying to describe a feeling. I can convince myself that I have expressed my fears this way, but the fear will remain within my field without sound expression.

Fear can be expressed in several ways; allowing the energy of it into your jaw to make your teeth chatter, allowing spontaneous weird sounds to emerge, or crying. Try putting your fingertips on your jaw, and (something I would recommend to newbies) massaging your jaw to the point where you can allow the fear to make your teeth and jaw "chatter" as though you are really cold. Sound is a key, of course, to go along with that; feeling for and allowing even the tiniest sound can open the door.

Expressing fear means giving in to it, allowing it up into the throat, into the voice, and then abandoning control and letting it happen. I nearly always feel better after I release, with more understanding of the triggering situation than before I started. This understanding does not always come immediately, or on the same day, but it does come.

With enough experience of expressing fear in sound, tears and body movement, fear will eventually evolve into trust over time in a given area or issue. As spoken of in Chapter 9, we all have an emotional backlog, and so fear about particular subjects cannot just necessarily evaporate with a couple of releases, though there are no rules.

Getting to fear "flashpoint" for the first time may be challenging. We have all developed intricate obstacle courses of resistance to fear expression. We have a lot of judgments running about how the fear will "swallow us", "it will be endless", "I will never survive it if I give into it", "I will just be creating more of it by focusing on it", etc. Those judgments need formal, sometimes repeated release. (See Part III, Chapter 17: "Judgment Release")

Taking Action Can Be Acting Out

Acting outwardly in the world to quell the feelings of fear inside, often in the form of desperately desiring to take immediate action of some sort is acting out the emotions instead of feeling them. All that does is delay the resolution of the fear, which will draw another situation to one's experience to be afraid about, another situation to trigger the same unreleased fear. In the long term, acting out emotions will not resolve them.

A woman worries that her son will contract the prostate cancer to which he is genetically predisposed. She spends significant energy trying to manage his health by giving him information and pressuring him to see a doctor. Some may say this is purely mother love. The woman's caring is certainly present in her motivation, but this is also worry taking action that reveals a terror, deeply buried, of her own mortality. She subconsciously fears death. When we have subconscious feelings, it is standard practice to project them onto someone else close to us because we do not always recognize that the feelings we are having are really ultimately about us. The person being projected onto is the mirror for what we cannot easily see about ourselves.

We all fear death to one extent or other, even if we do not consciously know it, because we have died many times before and we do not want to experience those feelings of being snuffed out again. Parts of our beings, the emotional, physical parts, hold encoded memories of these deaths buried deeply in the subconscious. These are parts of us that are not spirit. These parts do not rise to "heaven" between lives, and these parts have and hold the memory and terror of death.

Judgments on Expression

There are root judgments not only about what is feared but about daring to actually express the fear in pure, wordless sound. This sound might take the form of shrieks, keens, yelps, barks, crying out, tears, coughing, bodily shaking, quaking, chattering, or kriya jerking. A root judgment mentioned earlier that we all share is "If I dare allow this fear/terror to express through my body, I will go crazy/never survive it/create more of it/become dysfunctional". This fear and judgment of our own emotion of fear is barely even noticed anymore unless one gets close to considering releasing/expressing it in the sound and movement it would naturally like to make. And of course, if we do decide it's time to allow this emotion to express, we need to find safe space in which to express. Emotions do require a feeling and reality of safe space in order to fully let go in sound expression.

I have discovered that I cannot simply notice and accept my fear (or any emotion) with my mind/awareness or feeling bodies, and leave it at that. I have discovered I must take the additional step to express any triggered emotion to truly evolve them to the point where they can teach me what I need to know about how to heal, survive and live well, and change their macrocosmic, out-pictured reality on a mass scale.

Aspects of that big reality out there comprise a scary picture that feels overwhelming if we really feel it, but we can each do something about it to change it. However, most of us hold judgments that we cannot have any effect on the large-scale picture out there. What we can do is we can feel and EXPRESS what we feel about it all. Doing so can, does, and will help. The more of us who can dare to bring these emotions back inside ourselves through full acceptance of our emotional natures, which can be done by allowing ourselves to express emotions whenever triggered, starting now, the more help we can bring to the outer situation. The potential empowerment this can give each one of us is staggering.

It is the nature of emotions to express...and most of us were never taught that while growing up. We were taught the opposite in many overt and subtle ways. We were taught to hold them in. When we deny a part of ourselves, guilt and judgment shrink our expression. We disempower ourselves and therefore have less presence in any giving outward situation. As a result, we have a large reflection of this state of denial before us on the world stage, and we feel helpless to do anything about it. Expressing fear and any other held or triggered emotion helps to push guilt away from our energy field and literally grows our personal power.

"And It Has Come To Pass......"

And there were in the same country
weavers abiding, dreaming within,
about, and between themselves,
Spinning their moon-cloth webs by night;

And lo, the Mother of Song came upon them
and her music flowed round about them
awakening them gently as she sang thus unto
them:

You need never deny your fear
(nor yet your form) again
nor make of it a frozen prison
(nor a tomb),

For when embraced within the manger
of your unfolding, breathing desire,
your fear (along with your melting grief and
long-buried rage) becomes but
the cradle of your deepest truth,
calling you home to (and thru the birthing
process of) self-acceptance.

No external savior is needed, nor available,
only the birthing of your own true heart
thru self-forgiveness for having believed for so
long that so much that we feel, and are, is
unworthy of love, and, if damaged (as we all
are), incapable of reclamation, evolution,
transformation, resurrection; incapable

84

of sustaining (and indeed, becoming) the joyous
love, life, truth, and breath for which all that
we are has so long desired.

Behold, I sing and bring unto you
great tidings of great joy
For that which has long been hidden
shall now be unveiled, healed, and revealed;

For there is born to you this night,
in the city of the fore-mothers,
the spirit of truth, the longing,
that desire which is within you....

And this shall be a sign unto you:
You shall find her unfolding within a flowing
mantle of soft, strong, vibrant golden warmth
Dancing joyous circles of song within the heart;
yea, and within the womb, of this
Blessed Earth.

© Sara Mandal-Joy

Chapter 12: The Downside of (Held) Anger

The film "The Upside of Anger" features dramatic, familiar manifestations of acted-out rage: kicked down doors, sharp, blaming verbal exchanges, reckless driving, bodies striking bodies. We are also shown cold, expressionless, commanding rage delivered in others' faces, revenge fantasies wherein we witness an actor imagining horrible things happening to another and all manner of attempts to hold back the rage charge, preventing its escape. In the climactic moment, I fervently hoped that finally Hollywood was going to allow a full expression of primal sound to escape the main character's lips.

Alas, I was disappointed. We were instead shown the cinematic reflection of our society's refusal to "let the air out of the balloon through the original opening." What we did see trotted out were the usual clichés of what anger is and does. Emotions were allowed to subside and go back to sleep, with the occasional leaked tear. *Sigh.* At least no one pretended they were not angry! I imagined anger filling these metaphorical balloons of our emotional bodies to the bursting point, with the inevitable explosion bringing havoc and destruction instead of safe release and epiphany.

Individuals' Collective Rage Projected On the World Stage

We are all connected, not just in spirit, but in emotional essence as well. When we hold back our rage, the pressure added to the Big Balloon symbolizing humanity's collective rage intensifies somewhere else, through some "far distant" and weaker point in the "balloon skin", and then – POW!

Of course, the balloon forms again – weaker this time, more easily popped. When this "popping" occurs, someone gets hurt; sometimes us, sometimes "the other guy", who could be someone in another country, or on the streets in your own city. All over mainstream and alternative news alike, we watch the outer reflection of our inner collective anger in places like Iraq and Palestine, the Gulf of Mexico, and Syria, with new hotspots showing up regularly.

Not knowing what else to do with it, we shove our anger into others with blame, the rage being passed around, never evolving through appropriate expression.

We can imagine our rage is in such a balloon, and we are holding the balloon, two fingers clutching the cinched opening. Why wait for the bang and shreds when we could just let go? Letting go does not mean just sending it into the Earth or somewhere else through a technique; we have to take more responsibility than that, as our emotions are a part of us. Expressing anger in wordless sound "vibrates" the emotion, literally speeding it up, evolving it.

Once I've expressed and "opened" the area of compressed emotion, the light of truth can enter my emotional body in this area. At that point in my process I begin to glean very deep understandings about the roots of my anger. In part, I begin to see my involvement in a given situation, and I uncover what hidden awareness my held emotions had held back from surfacing. In most cases, I see and come to accept my responsibility in such triggering situations, in whatever way makes sense to me.

The part of me that is encased by or entwined with old anger has been shunted away in the dark for so long that it does not know what my mind and spirit know already. The vibration achieved through expression brings my angry parts up to speed. Ever notice that, having gone through an emotional time, you understand things much more deeply than before? That is emotional essence having caught up with the rest of the self.

This happens through a logical process. A part of the self previously held still is now vibrating via sound expression and therefore opening to the light of our spirits and minds, which then illuminates this emotional part of self, informing the Whole Self about the true nature of the problem.

Releasing Anger Safely and Effectively

Letting go means accepting and allowing the raw power of the rage that wants to just scream, stomp, smash or shout to have its way. Use a squishy pillow if necessary to block your sound, or a towel or cloth if you are on the road. However, anger can "prefer" unfettered sound expression in a safe space.

The anger that has built over the course of our lives can sometimes have been infused with violence, such as the physical abuse incurred as children being hit. When anger allowed to release back out of the self wants to stomp or smash things, allow this as much as possible while smashing things that do not mind being smashed, such as an old tree bough on the ground in the woods where no one can see or hear you. Doing so helps offload the old violence held in the body. Throw soft things around the room, pound your bed - whatever works to get you organically to the other side of the anger, when you feel a natural cycling down.

Additional rage release possibilities include jumping up and down and/or swinging your arms sharply up and down. Anger likes to sometimes "throw a tantrum", to use the terminology our parents and elders used against us growing up. Nowadays I realize that letting myself tantrum in private is an absolutely marvelous way of expressing primal rage.

Your body will communicate quite clearly, when you can allow this level of expression, what it really wants to do and how it really needs to express and how to move. Some people at certain times need to be able to smash breakable things. Buying a bunch of cheap pottery at yard sales and smashing it up safely in a room or garage when you get angry could satisfy the desire your rage might have to break things. Buying a heavy bag and some boxing gloves might satisfy the urge to hit with your body, getting the violence out in a safe and healthy way, preferably allowing sounds to emerge all the while.

It can be helpful to formally intend, ahead of being triggered and also perhaps once triggered but not having moved yet, to allow your sound to come up once your body is in motion. Then, once Body has engaged, have a spot of awareness if you can to open to sound coming forth. The moment of "impact" can be a great moment to simultaneously let out a short or long bellow. If the bellow comes naturally, let it take you over, even if you are scared about it taking you to some place you will never recover from and even if/when judgments swim up spontaneously. Be sure to release these judgments when your sound dies back...these are the times the judgments can be most effectively released (see Part III, the Judgment Release chapter). Even "faking it until you make it" in terms of bellowing when you use your physical force can eventually connect you to real, organic sound.

Any hard, yang, physical movement can activate your true rage sound. I also have spent a lot of time in parked cars at the edges of big parking lots with the windows rolled up, even on 90 degree days, slamming rolled up towels off the dashboard and hitting the steering wheel with my open palms. This works well when no other safe space is available. Once the sound starts to come forth, no matter what you do to get it going, the stopper will be off and it gets easier from there until you will have no trouble whatsoever letting your rage move freely.

Feared Repercussions

Sometimes subconscious terror of repercussions for moving rage in pure loud sound has got a vice-grip on anger's organic expression. Another way in, therefore, can be to focus on releasing judgments of what will happen to you (or how "bad" you are, according to internalized judgments) if you were to allow loud, brash sound to come out when you are angry (even if your mind knows you are in safe space sound wise). If this is the case, start first by moving the fear that is holding down the rage. Fear and anger have a symbiotic relationship and can often be holding one another down, attempting with all subconscious might to keep the lid on. It is possible to start by moving fear, then allowing yourself to flip to anger if that is what arises in the moment. You can then flip back to fear or move some combination of "terrorage" (a feeling of both emotions mixed together) until you feel complete.

When you dare to release your anger this way, you are helping undo the mass of denied and inappropriately-expressed rage across the planet, directly affecting volatile situations in war-torn areas of the world. If need be, release the judgment that this could not be true. Every time we allow angry feelings to release safely in pure sound, it "goes out the hole" and eases the pressure on the Whole.

Chapter 13: Proactive Vs. Reactive Healing

It is very important to allow yourself to respond to safe, proactive triggers, (as well as the scary, reactive ones) so that it is not always life's hardships in your face that put you through your paces. I have made tapes of triggering music and with burning candles and prayer, I have triggered the pain I knew was lurking and impacting on my life every day. When at all possible I set aside whatever I am doing to deal with what is rising emotionally in me. I have found that, in the long run, this commitment to putting my healing first results in fewer harsh setbacks in my outer reality than I used to have.

Surrender to what rises in you with as little control as possible on its expression. Proactively dealing with your emotions as they are triggered means taking advantage of every nuance of emotion where you have a sense that the emotion could be expressed and released if you simply focus on it for a short time. The willingness to pay complete attention to the emotion you really feel in the moment helps it to emerge all the way to the surface for ignition, expression and release.

A "Safe" Trigger: Allowing Fantasy To Trigger Proactively

My friend Carmen wanted more information about releasing fear. She asked for an example based on a fear she had about losing her freedom in the form of money (Carmen and her partner are heavily invested in the stock market). I painted for her the following fantasy:

Imagine a stock market crash. You stand to lose thousands of dollars with slim hope of recovery. In six months you will have difficulty paying your mortgage, unthinkable only a short while ago. You must radically change your lifestyle, which looks like a severe cutback in your freedom.

Your days become filled with fear. If you are observant of your body's responses and honest with yourself, you recognize the fear in your solar plexus region, maybe your jaw. You might even have a headache, feel intermittently nauseous or lightheaded. You start to feel "delicate" and uncomfortably vulnerable.

Imagining such a fear picture can activate fear in your body as if it were really happening. This would be what I call a "safe trigger", since this scene is only imagined, not really manifesting in your life. I did not suggest to Carmen, nor would I to anyone, to fantasize negatively on purpose to bring up these triggers. As she mentioned, the fear was already within her and she was aware of it. These types of fear pictures arising from the fear hidden within can come unbidden, from within or without (say, from a friend). At the time of noticing the fantasy, feeling into one's fear in response can constitute a safe trigger scenario.

Another definition of a "safe trigger" is when you fear something is sure to happen or about to happen, and you feel and express that fear in advance of anything "bad" happening, then the feared outcome does not manifest and turns out to be nothing but a good trigger.

Reactive or "Unsafe" Triggers

A manifestation that brings an actual reversal to your fortunes monetarily or otherwise would be an "unsafe trigger". Manifesting a lot of unsafe triggers indicates that you have ignored one too many previous, lesser-magnitude fear triggers. In my example, the unsafe trigger would be where you actually get seriously reversed financially in order to overcome your repeatedly reinforced resistance to feeling and expressing your fear. The trigger is drawn, or magnetized as an experience in order to wake you up in that area. You had become too numb or too resistant to experience anything of lesser magnitude getting you off the dime emotionally.

What is the Payoff?

"But what do I do with the fears when they arise? It is so hard not to try to think about or do something else to take my mind off it all, so I do not have to feel this fear anymore," Carmen said.

She has arrived now at a "choice-point". She is free to distract herself from that fearful undercurrent with various means at her disposal. This is denial of how she really feels.

Feeling hard emotions is not easy. She wants to deny that she is afraid by overlaying activities or new thoughts that cover up the fear so she does not have to notice anymore that she is afraid. For Carmen, faith must be cultivated that there will be some sort of payoff in the end that will be worth going through the feelings all the way to the other side.

When they occur spontaneously, imagined scenarios are good for triggering old fear. They cause the physio-emotional system to respond no differently at root than if the feared event had manifested. Our collective judgments have resulted in grooved habit patterns that encourage focusing on something else to stimulate a more pleasurable emotional response. These judgments say something to the effect of "I am causing unnecessary fear with such thoughts".

Again, I am not suggesting intentionally generating fearful thoughts. Simply notice when the thoughts arise organically. Once you have noticed them, you may start to feel afraid as the thoughts begin to flesh out. This fear can be expressed in sound or tears (see Chapter 11 for fuller details on releasing fear as an emotion). The more willing and able we are to vibrate (express) emotions with smaller triggers the more safe or "proactive" triggers we will experience as opposed to unsafe or "reactive" triggers.

Chapter 14: Recognizing and Releasing Guilt

Some people think that guilt is useful. There exists a judgment in the collective subconscious that says we would run amok, indulging every impulse, no matter how inappropriate, if we did not have "healthy guilt" (now there is a contradiction in terms) to keep us in check. Nonsense! Were we truly healthy, our free will choices and actions would flow freely, even impulsively, yet harm none. Guilt is not a tool or an emotion. It is not our "conscience" telling us we just did something wrong and now we need to feel bad about it. It takes up energetic space where emotional response is supposed to be.

Moving from a guilt-ridden state to a healed one is a process, and in an environment where free will is encouraged, there will be mistakes along the journey to attaining balance. Using guilt to keep us in line has not served humankind, for there can be no self-acceptance of all the facets of ourselves if guilt is in charge.

Guilt is really just empty space. It is lack of vibration and emotional expression. Guilt makes our energy shrink, mutes our capacity to respond truthfully and dims our awareness in any situation. Guilt keeps us far from the truth. When guilt is present you cannot know yourself fully or know what is happening around you, and others cannot get to know you fully.

Recognizing Guilt's Voice

There is no loving understanding in the voice of guilt. It can sound right intellectually, but feels wrong to our emotional body. Guilt takes a kernel of truth and uses it against us with a hurtful twist. This unloving tone is one way to recognize its presence, especially if we are chronically swamped in guilt. Over time, as we have learned to habitually deny our deep emotional responses to triggers, we have made room for guilt and we have lost sensitivity to be able to always tell the difference between guilt and love.

Guilt divides us by turning parts of ourselves against the rest, in turn separating us from Spirit and each other, triggering hopelessness and a sense of futility which leads to depression, addiction, and other chronic nasties. Guilt uses hindsight against us, saying we should have known because of XYZ, we should have done this, we were wrong not to do that. Its voice can disguise itself, often "reflected" to us from others outside us wagging subtly and overtly disapproving fingers our way. If guilt is synthesized down to its most basic message, it is saying we should be doing better than we already are. If self-acceptance is the key to healing, guilt is utter lack of self-acceptance, and is in and of itself a hindrance to the healing process.

An over-abundance of guilt in my energy field draws punishment to me, because I am most likely believing the message that I have done wrong and need to "learn a lesson". The more I can vibrate my emotions, thereby removing guilt from my energy field, the fewer punishing reflections I will encounter from outside me.

Awareness of Guilt Leads to Healing and Dealing

Guilt's presence, however, is a signpost that buried emotion lies hidden underneath it, and this emotion can be noticed, and ideally, subsequently expressed and released. I need to notice how I really feel when guilt's voice speaks to me, and then give into that emotional response, not just in words, but in sound and tears, in a safe space. When authentic response is given to every stimulus, as fully as possible, the space for guilt to stay or enter closes and one's personal will becomes freer over time as a result.

Guilt is not living essence, and as a result, cannot vibrate along with the emotional wells it is sitting on. When emotions that had been previously surrounded or suppressed with a layer of guilt begin to express and vibrate, guilt floats off. We only notice this by becoming aware after the fact that we no longer feel guilty about a certain confluence of events or stimuli that would have previously triggered a guilty response.

Guilt's Other Face: Blame

Conversely, the more I deny my true response to emotional triggers, the more guilt enters the space and speaks to me from outside and inside myself. In the worst-case scenario, guilt runs my life. When guilt is projected outward onto another person or situation, it comes out in the form of blame. If I find myself blaming another, or others blaming me, it can usually be traced back to guilt, either theirs, or mine reflected to me by them, or both.

For example, let's say my partner has a defensive response when I ask her whether she mailed off the letters we agreed needed to go out today. She listed the reasons why she could not get to it and clearly was feeling as though she had done something wrong. She was angry and defensive with me on the surface for bringing it up; underneath, she was angry at her own guilt that was already telling her how wrong she was to have not mailed the important letters on time.

When I am in touch with my true feelings underneath guilt, I can feel and notice the sadness/grief, anger/rage or fear/terror I may be triggering in another. Loving intent wants harmony. The more I feel and express my own emotions, the more I can feel love for and have loving presence with other people. I can then follow true inner guidance to bring harmony and love back to our surrounding world.

Noticing and acknowledging guilt is the responsible first step in disarmament during any personal war, and as mentioned, can then be released with the true expression of the emotions it conceals. The more we can disarm and own our sides of our personal vendettas, the more we as individuals, the microcosm of the planet itself, can disempower warmongering on the large scale.

Chapter 15: Emotions and Functionality

Many people, when considering stepping onto an emotional healing path face the fear or judgment that if we all gave into our emotions, nobody would be functional or get anything done that needs to be done.

This is a very common fear, or judgment. Yet, the emotional body is smarter than we give her credit for. She knows how to get the job done, and often draws the triggers when there is space and time to move them. Not always, but a lot more than one would realize, if the possibilities were allowed and tried and some time and deeds accrued.

Judgments on Free Expression of Emotions

In part, the judgment says if people who are chronically suppressing (i.e. the majority of the population) receive triggers and allow themselves to express emotionally, these people would be instantly incapacitated for an indefinite length of time. Moreover, this would happen to everyone at once, with bedlam and societal crash resulting. The reality is that not everyone is going to allow their expression to come up all at once, all at the same time.

Another way to word the judgment is, if we all let ourselves express our feelings, anarchy and chaos would result. This is a judgment on emotions, and includes these nested sub-judgments within:

Chaos is bad.

Chaos, even temporary chaos, will result in harm to myself or others.

It is safer to repress expression rather than allow it.

Denial works better than allowance of emotional expression.

Denial allows for more functional humans. (This last one I think could be a "truth" in the short run, but watch out for those negative reversals of fortune you do not see coming, as the denial catches up with you... BAM!)

I can fully release these judgments and allow these emotions to express responsibly, ideally with myself in a safe space. The more I do this process of judgment release (see Chapter 11) and safe emotional release, the more I re-define what emotions are: a natural human vibration dealt with responsibly that helps create harmony and increase love.

Not Everyone Releases At Once

My experience of being in groups, even groups of "movers", i.e. those expressing or "moving" emotions freely and appropriately, is that there is nearly always someone not moving, someone who could "take over" whatever function needs to be taken over. Additionally, if I have a job to do, and I am in the midst of doing it, I do not often find myself triggered to the point of needing to let go of my function entirely; i.e. receiving such a massive trigger that my essential function is going to need a replacement. There are exceptions, and if it does happen, often an organic replacement scenario emerges.

Nevertheless, there can be times when I absolutely need to postpone the emotional release for later, with a strong willing intent to really get back to it as soon as possible and not deny it further by letting it slide back into unconsciousness. Cultivating this intent to heal and deal asap, the trigger can often be accessed even hours later within safe sound space.

If you do find yourself letting the trigger slide for days without returning, beating yourself up for it won't help. Starting in this moment, going forward, you can notice without judgment if the slide is rooted in a habit of placing the emotions as second or last priority. Delaying dealing with your triggers can source from unexamined fear of your own hidden emotions, alongside the judgment bed we have been discussing.

Like any other developed skill, practice and more experience helps. My expressive intention gets a boost when I have proof that my life often improves in quality from a practice of emotional release. I then am more inclined to release more feelings as they are triggered, in a timely way. This can be like a positive feedback loop. I then develop and hone my vigilance to change my habits of denial and place emotional healing in the forefront.

Releasing In The Midst of a Busy Day

I can move gently/subtly (like teeth chattering, low moaning or grrrr'ing) and sometimes continue what I am doing. I have driven many safe miles, for example, while simultaneously moving pretty big. My body knows how to do it. I am not saying everyone's does; it takes some experience.

When I worked in the software industry, I would get triggered at work, and then step away from my desk for a spontaneous break (or as soon as possible), go out in my car, drive to a corner of the parking lot, and let it out. If it was too hot for that (which was rarely; I did not mind feeling overheated, it somehow seemed appropriate), or somehow felt unsafe, I would go into a patch of woods. I would take out even something as small as a hankie, or a hand towel, or take a layer of clothing, and express into that. You might be surprised how much sound gets blocked. Ideally, emotions want a safe place for expression, where they really KNOW they will not be heard or stopped.

There are creative alternatives, if the emotional body is put "first". I will drop most things I am doing, once I know I am triggered, to find a modicum of safe space and time to express what comes up for me.

Walking The Fog

We have discussed the feared impact on continued functionality of weaving emotional expression into our busy day, but what about the times when we cannot express anything at all, even if we want to?

Deep autumn is a classic time of year for the pea soup of depression to hit. In the Pacific Northwest, the rains kick in as the sun becomes a fleeting memory, and all the things I have been running from for months begin to creep forward into my consciousness, pushing for triggering and release. If I have not "cleaned house" in a while, these ghosts emerging from the depths of my closet have the ability to overwhelm me - and in so doing I become, like my backyard, heavy and laden with muck, mist and bog, and I find I cannot move as easily.

Most of us know what real depression looks and feels like. Even if we have not experienced a depressive period ourselves, we probably each know or have heard about somebody who has, and how they were during it.

Depression is rife with a feeling that there is no way to get out from under, that nothing can work. A time of depression is a time where we look at life through shit-colored glasses. There is no energy to do the things we like to do or have to do. The life force drained out, we vegetate, flatline. We feel squashed and compressed. We cannot feel. We are not functional, but not because we are being too expressive; instead, we cannot express much of anything. We indulge in distractions and addictions of various kinds. We are uncomfortably numb.

The root of depression is accumulated, unexpressed and denied emotions. Having an overabundance of old emotions in one's energy field decreases the energy level and contributes to low self-esteem and lack of self-care. All of this combines to create body imbalance and generalized hopelessness that can build in a vicious cycle.

It can be very uncomfortable for the loved ones of a depressed individual (DI) to be around him or her, and the kneejerk tendency is to help them lift out of it any way possible. They try to distract the DI from what ails them (should that even be evident), point out how so-and-so from Iraq or Syria or Palestine has it worse so buck up, become an ad hoc salesperson for the latest miracle pharmaceutical or toss a few hope ropes in case the DI has the strength or ability to grab one and hoist themselves up.

Realistically, there is nothing a friend of a DI can do that is more effective than staying close by while the DI muddles through as best s/he can, ready to lend a helping hand when asked. For the DI, it is a time to find as many mental judgments about his/her situation that can be found, and then formally release them out loud (e.g. "I release the judgment that I am never going to have the life I want," etc.). Sometimes doing this can trigger the tears, rages or freakouts that can dispel the heavy fog.

Whenever I am depressed, what also helps me find my way through is getting into my body. If I can walk a little, do some deep breathing, yoga, Somatics, anything to help me focus inward – it can enable me to get into some sound expression, which always helps shift me when nothing is moving. Inertia begets depression begets more inertia. Distraction and medication can be very short-term solutions that in the end reveal themselves as circular train trips returning us to the very station we try to escape.

All of this can be beside the point if one is deemed clinically depressed. If this is the case, no suggestion here may be appropriate for those who may feel they require medication for a short- or long-term period to help them function at all.

Hating or pressuring myself to pick myself up by my bootstraps does not work either, but is rather another circumnavigation. Sometimes, temporarily, nothing at all works. The best I can do is sit for a while in the low vibration of hopelessness with what is happening or not happening, accepting myself as best I can for being in this place, trusting on the way to trust that this too shall pass.

* * * * * * * *

Part III

The Mental Body

Chapter 16: Proactive Thinking and The Great God of Logic

"I am in such a fog today." "If I only had a brain." "...brain fart" ...these are some of the ways some of us have described our state of affairs when we feel our mental bodies to be dysfunctional. How does one heal a mind? First off, who really knows what the mind is? Is mind the same as the brain? Or is the mental body our thoughts? A crucible for making decisions? A psychic radio, tuning in strong, clear signals and homing in on weak ones? Our own private study? How private is this study, anyhow?

I would say the mental body is a halfway house, the balance point between our Spirit and our emotional and physical bodies. It receives input coming up from "below" (physical/emotional) and "above" (Spirit....see Part IV for discussion) and synthesizes that input, hopefully into something cohesive.

The Mental Body's Disconnected State

Thinking is often driven by churning, unnoticed emotions. When emotions in this state can be expressed, they do not churn thoughts as much, and both mind and will (i.e. the emotional body) can rest. A healing mind with emotions at rest might look more like a sensitive version of *Star Trek's* Mr. Spock, offering information and its considered opinion when asked, but otherwise staying behind the scenes. To his credit, Spock never took over, he never initiated the action; he waited to be asked. It seemed as though he had usually considered all the angles, because seemingly he had all the information at his disposal. But without a vibrating will, (since for him, emotions were not logical and were therefore banned from his awareness as best he could) his decisions were too mental, therefore too rigid. He didn't really have the whole picture.

Our mental body's downfall in its unhealed state is its disconnect from the rest of the self. Through damage or trauma, our spiritual essence, our "I-ness", the part we identify as "Me", does not descend all the way into our physical and emotional bodies. It merely has a toe dipped in those waters, and lodges some of itself in the mind, leaving its majority floating somewhere just outside the Self. Similarly, if one is not connecting to their emotions, the mind has no way of gleaning input from the feelings.

Without spirit and will (emotions) fully integrated into the emotional and physical, the "road" leading to our halfway house is in such shoddy repair that in many cases it is undriveable, impassible. There is no flow of information from the emotional and physical bodies to the mental body, so mind does not have all the information, only what has worked or not worked in the past. Thus it is inevitably trapped in the same space that Spock's great mind was trapped: in the seductive vice-grip of The Great God of Logic.

Getting Physical Helps The Mental

Physical activity such as dancing or hiking can help draw the spiritual and mental bodies into closer contact with the physical and emotional. Intuition and spontaneous visions become unlocked as the mental and spiritual bodies "descend" into corporeal reality. Ever notice how much more alive and clear your thoughts and visions become at various moments while receiving a bodywork session? Integration is happening; the "road" is being repaired, information transfer is being restored between emotions, body, and mind. Emotional expression as described in other sections of this book is the final step that is often missed here, as physical activity alone won't complete the repair.

Stretching, yoga, bodywork (either on one's self or via a practitioner), cardiovascular exercise and Somatics exercises help deepen breathing and help the whole system slow down. This kind of physical activity especially helps slow the mind and its whirling thoughts, by helping spirit descend more into Body. When the spiritual body is fully integrated with the physical, and emotions are being noticed and felt, mind becomes more fully embodied as well, and enters the "Now Moment". Habitually, our mental bodies like to take off into the past or future, and at those times, we are not fully present.

Getting Emotional Helps The Mental

When we are "in our heads" we need to take time to express feelings that are lurking just under the surface. Some signals that indicate that feelings are rising to the surface include trying to figure stuff out, having conversations in our heads with other people, or fantasizing how we wish things would have worked out better than they did.

Whenever I am feeling mentally spinny, I close my eyes, take a few deep, slow, full breaths and feel into myself to determine whether some emotion is present that needs to move. Nearly always at these times, I do need to move emotions. After movement, my thoughts slow down, the road between my mental and emotional bodies becomes ploughed and my inner Spock can take his rightful role, connecting Spirit visionary clarity with gut feelings, also known as intuition.

Heart As the Balance Point

What is happening at an electromagnetic level is that my spirit, instead of floating just outside my Self as described earlier is now magnetized toward the rest of me after I have expressed myself emotionally. This is because after I have expressed my emotions, they vibrate faster and thus emit a stronger, steadier, more coherent magnetic charge to 'hold' spirit present. When this happens, mind can form the perfect balance point between the two and spirit and emotions can meet there. Bonds of simpatico and understanding are formed. It is in this space when mind can become one with true heart.

Relational bonds are formed on the inner, which can then reflect in my outer experience as heart bonding occurring with another; the meeting of the minds. The direction of flow is inside of me → outside of me. When I balance with myself as a result of my spirit receiving my emotional body's expression, I form these heart bonds and develop self-love. Without these inner bonds, I cannot truly love and bond with another.

When my emotions, usually sourcing in my lower three chakras are activated and vibrating, they draw my spiritual energy from the upper chakras and beyond down towards the heart. Electromagnetic balance within the Self is found in the center point or heart.

Prior to emotional expression my receptive centers in my emotional body are full up and not generating as much magnetism toward my spirit, so my spirit is literally floating away and my point of awareness is drawn up into my head.

The role of judgments, also known as belief structures and expectations, are like walls that compartmentalize and narrow the mind, and this is the main area in which the mental body needs healing. We will discuss the role of judgments in the next section.

Chapter 17: Judgment Release

A wise teacher (actually, my partner Bee) once said to me that words are like spells; they can work their magic for or against us. In this context, only a fool says that talk is cheap. The actual cost of pronouncements and the kind of generalities that pepper everyday conversation can be, in fact, quite astronomical. To painfully extend the metaphor, we can find ourselves paying "interest" for many years, never touching the principal.

What are judgments? One way to see them are as labels that become beliefs. A second way could be stuck layers of emotional energy translated by the mental body. A judgment is a preconception about something. Through the lens of judgment, something or someone is seen as "good," "bad," "right," "wrong." The end result comprises a distortion. We think we know a person, place, thing or situation without having to get to know it or feel it for what it really is in the moment.

Thus, judgments compose barriers to relating to something and stop us from having a dynamic relationship with that something or someone. Judgments, spoken or thought, are ways we cast spells on ourselves. They are one of the mental body's coping mechanisms for dealing with overwhelming realities. They give us the illusion of control by making rules or stating the way a situation, person, place, or thing IS. The hidden cost of making judgments is that they become a "thought form" - a rigid structure in the mind that can magnetize and recreate unpleasant situations that match the judgment's rules and expectations, narrowing the openings for epiphany.

We run the danger of re-conditioning ourselves every time we reiterate a judgment we have been holding, both in casual conversation and emotional diatribe. Acting out an emotion instead of expressing it at the root level in sound or body movement is the problem here while stating judgments as truths. When we are ranting, if we are not ranting with an intention to reveal the deeper emotional content for full release, we are in danger of seating the judgments within the rant even more deeply than before. Ranting itself is a good path toward full wordless release, but if one chronically stops the process after ranting and rarely or never descends into the full ignition of non-verbal expression, judgments can solidify, forming damaging clutter in one's energy field.

Right Rather Than Happy

Parts of us would rather be right than happy. We have lost awareness of how powerful our expectations and judgments are; how they shape the realities and experiences that "come toward us from the future". We have also lost awareness of the intense emotions just under the surface, often powering the judgment's need to be right. To complete the cycle, judgments also empower denial of emotional realities within us. Even though we lose when a judgment we have been holding seems to prove itself true, there is a "perverse deliciousness" in the satisfaction of saying 'I knew this would happen!', and the mental body trumps the emotional...again. This grooved pattern of reaching for the "reward" of being right rather than reaching for deeper truth is one of the main areas in the mental body that needs to change if healing is to happen.

The more I heal and deal and practice becoming aware of my judgments for what they are, the easier judgments are to spot. I can start with the big obvious judgments in my life and begin to notice how the subtler ones reveal themselves. I can recognize that a part of me believes or thinks this, and in addition to the release process, my greater Self needs to find compassion for the part of my mind that thinks this, because that part isn't wrong. It was merely a way this part of me had coped with a particular reality in the past, when it didn't have the proper awareness or tools to get the awareness.

Verbal Judgment Release

Clearing judgments can allow me to see a situation anew in the moment, and in doing so, I can reinvent my reality as it manifests before my eyes. A good way to release mental body judgments is by stating such a release out loud -- the antidote to the "spell" I put on myself when I originally made the judgment.

With as much emotional presence as you can muster, say something like "I release the judgment that..." and then name the judgment you have been holding, e.g. "...Rottweilers are dangerous". Then look for the judgments that support the one you just let go. "I release the judgment that dogs are only safe on leashes. I forgive myself for having believed that animals do not like me. I allow the belief to dissolve that the world is frightening. I let go now of the belief that I can never feel safe.

What often happens during this exercise of releasing judgments out loud is that more and deeper emotions will be revealed and triggered to the surface.

Releasing judgments can trigger emotional release, and conversely, emotional release can trigger the awareness of more root-level judgments.

Verbal, out-loud releasing of judgments is crucial in assisting oneself to stay present in the here and now.

Internal Judgment Release

In addition to external judgment release via the spoken form, most of us have made judgments internally and need to then release these judgments within our minds. The same methodology applies, only silently. These internal releases are most effective while already emoting, when judgments relating to the emotions being expressed swim up to conscious awareness in the moment. It is not helpful to interrupt emotional expression in order to speak the release of judgments, so instead you can release expression of the judgment internally. I would recommend waiting until any given emotional release layer has completed before releasing further judgments verbally – in other words, don't interrupt your emotional flow in order to speak words. You can wait until you "come up for air", and then more judgments you've discovered can be released out loud.

Internal releases are not substitutes for the external ones, but necessary corollaries. Realistically, they are of secondary importance relative to spoken judgment releases. Still, internal or silent judgment release can be helpful and effective for identifying key judgments and rounding out the approach toward supporting our true need to free and heal ourselves from the confines of belief structures.

Judgment "Nests"

Use any wording for the form of your judgment release that feels right to you in the moment. Notice that as you follow the trail of judgments, they tend to get deeper and more to the core of the root judgments you hold. These are the kind of deep beliefs that imprinted our psyche at the dawn of our awareness, and continue to cut across many arenas of our existence to this day.

Pay attention inside, as you sift through a particular nest of judgments during their verbal release, for the emotions underneath that may start to stir and move. Allow as much emotional release as you feel you can in whatever ways you can. Releasing judgments and the hidden emotions powering them can allow you to view a situation with fresh eyes, seeing and accepting it for what it is now. Cultivate the art of speaking specifically rather than generally, e.g. "I got attacked by a Rottweiler when I was ten, and I have felt afraid of them up to now" instead of "dogs are dangerous and scary." Play with releasing as many beliefs as you can find -- do a little ceremony if you like -- and dare to release the judgment that this process could not work for you, is bullshit, and that you would rather be right than happy!

I have come to recognize how I judge constantly, something every one of us does every day. Practicing judgment release has raised my level of awareness of how much I judge. Doing so allows me to take greater responsibility for what happens to me. Formally releasing judgments may feel awkward and self-conscious at first, but the results can be truly magic.

The things and people I judge often are "forced" to appear to me as though satisfying the judgments, i.e. making the judgments appear as though they were truths and the ensuing experiences the proof. This is primarily because the underlying locked-in emotions are magnetic.

They hold the judgment in place while magnetizing experiences that repeat the original experience with the twist the thought form has placed on it.

Thus, psychically, once the judgments or thought-forms were put into place in my awareness, further experiences seem to have to conform to the existence of the judgment. That means that when I originally decided what something or someone was, I created a pattern that energetically began to attract its exact match. I have not realized that I am holding the judgment in my mental body from long ago, outside memory, when I made the judgment in order to cope with an overwhelming reality.

When I can release the judgment and heal the emotion underneath, its drawing power is decreased or eliminated, and further experiences that have previously "satisfied" the judgment's validity are no longer necessary. Depending on the strength and intensity of the judgment or judgment "nest", the release or a particular judgment can be a one-time-only necessity, or there may need to be several iterations of the same judgment release, along with the release of its accompanying emotion that become entangled with it, in order to eliminate further experiences reflecting the judgment.

An example of the pattern is reflected in the following story. Ellen, a woman who dreams of singing on stage, holds judgments on herself that she is not good at singing, that her voice is weak, that others are far better performers and vocalists than she is. After taking some singing lessons for a couple years and singing along to songs on the radio, she begins to tentatively "put herself out there" at open mikes, singing along with her guitar or with someone else's accompaniment.

One night, sitting at a table at her favorite open mike event, she is listening to someone else doing their set but can't help overhearing two men talking at a table nearby about wanting a female singer for their new band.

She begins to tune into their conversation, and hears her name mentioned by one of them as a possibility. "No way," his friend responds. "We need someone with a strong voice, and also Ellen is way too reined in when she performs, have you watched her up there? We need someone who's really going to hold the audience's attention in more ways than one."

Ellen is horrified and ashamed, and ends up leaving early. When she goes home, she allows herself to deal with her triggered emotions and cries long and loud in the privacy of her own room. Her feelings begin with the shame and self-loathing that are on the surface. At certain points the feelings shift, touching on anger at the men, anger at herself for "not being good enough" and fear that they, and she, have been "right all along". Strange sounds and huge volume roll out of her, surprising her a bit at their intensity.

When her expression quiets after a while, she blows her nose, gulps a bit and says out loud, with feeling, "I forgive myself for having believed for so long that I have a shitty singing voice! I release the judgment that I am not good enough to sing in front of a band or in front of any audience! I no longer believe that I am not captivating enough of a singer and performer to hold anyone's attention onstage!" She keeps noticing new judgments popping up as the old ones are voiced, and keeps releasing every judgment out loud that come to mind. These judgments seem to rise to awareness one after another during her release process, like pearls on a string, so she just keeps going and releasing each one in case they're all judgments and not truths about how and who she really is.

A month goes by. At a different open mike, Sheila, a woman whose stage chops on guitar and voice Ellen has long admired approaches Ellen after Ellen's set. Ellen has been thrilled at how much better her singing has felt of late, finding nuances and supple strength in her voice that she hadn't previously noticed. Sheila lets Ellen know she is starting a women's singing collective, with long-term intent to perform original songs, and would Ellen be interested in being a part of it? Ellen eagerly agrees to the offer and six months later is part of a tight, well-liked and well-known local quartet of female performers, receiving regular audience appreciation and cultivating a growing, calm, strengthening sense of inner fulfillment.

Like Ellen, sometimes I will follow the "trail" of judgments that start with the surface judgment, such as "I release the judgment that my father does not want to know me as I am", with an intent to get to the core judgment(s) underneath:

→ "I forgive myself for having believed for so long that Dad really hates me"

→ "I forgive myself for having believed for so long that fathers hate sons who do not follow in their footsteps"

→ "I forgive myself for having believed for so long that God is not there for me."

→ "I forgive myself for having believed for so long that God hates me"

→ "I forgive myself for having believed for so long that God does not want to know me"

→ "I choose to release the judgment that I am not worthy of support, that I am bad, that I am not okay as I am, that I am wrong to exist as the real me"

You can see how "core" this can get. Sometimes following the judgment trail does bring up some old feelings that are in essence wrapped around the thought-forms (i.e. formations made of thoughts, which become obstacles to light and true understanding), which ideally need to be released in the moment they are triggered by the judgment release process, as Ellen did in our previous example. The emotions entwined with the judgments need release when triggered in order for my mental body to fully release my judgments at the deepest levels.

I actually practiced these particular judgment releases and ensuing emotional release about fathers, sons and God as described, and after some time passed, the relationship with my own father transformed rather naturally and dramatically from one of distance and enmity to closeness and restored love. As a result of doing this work, reality shifts in my own life have been proven, and not just in this example, to be more than a theoretical or hit'n'miss exercise.

One final example - let us say I just had an encounter with a policeman who threatened to come and throw me in jail. I retreat to my safe space and I start to release terror in sound. When I feel ready to talk again, I begin to release these judgments, as forcefully as I can: "I release the judgment that I hate police. I release the judgment that I always lose to authority. I release the judgment that I cannot win. I reject the judgment that the powers that be will always rule my life. I release the judgment that I can never step out of line. I forgive myself for believing that I am powerless." Judgments released powerfully out loud with strong intent to let them go combined with emotional movement is a very effective tool for freeing the mental and emotional bodies.

Truth vs. FLATs

An ancient, deeply ingrained judgment can often feel to us like a truth, but we release it anyway, because one cannot release truth. When the judgments have cleared, truth is all that is left, and it flows naturally. Over time, FLAT judgments like these (i.e. those that F.eel L.ike A T.ruth) need repeated release to get all of them out of our mental bodies.

How can one tell the difference between a truth and a FLAT judgment? Try to feel deeply whether the FLAT feels good to you, or if it has the resonance of a "grim reality we each have to deal with". Truth usually feels good and is not something we need to manipulate ourselves or other people to accept. We usually have some trapped emotional energy around FLATs that we can notice if we look.

FLATs are usually so deeply ingrained and have been so repeatedly conditioned into our pictures of reality that one release doesn't seem to do much. I can sometimes have an inner response to a FLAT judgment release that goes something like "yeah, right", as though I am voicing an untrue affirmation, something the rest of me believes it knows is B.S. In this case, suspect that there is indeed hidden charge embedded with the FLAT.

Judgment release in any given judgment bed can often be a lengthy, iterative process, but we must start somewhere. Dedication to the process over time helps us doggedly keep releasing the same one every time we notice the judgment proving itself in our reality. Beware any tendency to give in to *another* overarching belief that judgment release doesn't work or "I wouldn't be having this happen again". We have in many cases been pounding these judgments into ourselves for lifetimes, and it's going to take some work over time to move certain judgments fully out of ourselves.

The Inverted Pyramid

A friend once said the judgments or belief systems and structures we each hold are like marbles in an inverted pyramid. You have to take out the top layers of marbles first, then follow the trail down the layers to the bottom-most marble. You cannot just go to the bottom ones first and remove them, because they are holding up a whole structure of beliefs. This is why searching for and releasing a whole string of nested judgments can be helpful, because one judgment often leads to the next.

Those bottom marbles, or core judgments, are the FLAT ones, with all the weight of unprocessed judgment "marbles" layered on top. As stated, those core judgments have to sometimes be released again and again, whenever noticed, while noticing and releasing all the ones they are holding up too.

Sometimes I notice that I will release the same judgment over and over and it still seems to manifest physically in my life, and I still seem to believe it. These FLATs are not only supporting other higher-layer judgments, but are also entrapped with fear, grief and rage way down deep in our emotional bodies, as depicted in Ellen's story above. This intertwining with old held emotions is what holds judgments present despite repeated attempts to release them out loud verbally. The judgment release I am doing out loud is of value insofar as it's making me aware that I am still holding it, and at some level remain impacted by it.

Some Classic Judgments on Anger and Fear

If my terror release flips suddenly to a rage release, I might, when I am done my sounding or pounding of pillows or whatever safe release I am doing in my own space, release judgments such as:
→ I cannot tolerate limits
→ I will always rebel
→ I always end up in battle with authority
→ Authority is always wrong
→ I always lose
→ There has to be a winner and a loser

→ They are always wrong
→ I have to be right
→ If I am wrong, I die
→ If I am right, I survive
→ If I'm right I'm happy
→ There has to be battle in order to overturn the status quo

Like judgments on anything else, judgments of my fear and judgments of what is feared can be formally and verbally released out loud. This is very effective in removing the "denial stopper corks" from our bottled-up energy. State with as much realness as you can:

→ I release the judgment that if I give in to my fear, it will never end.
→ I release the judgment that if I express my fear in sound, I will become crazy.
→ I release the judgment that expressing fear through my body is just plain wrong.

These are some examples of widely held consensus beliefs about fear that can be released verbally out loud in formal statements just as I have described. There are many more. The out-loud releasing undoes the magic spells in our minds that we have woven with our prior decrees about fear. Releasing judgments about fear also helps normalize fear as just another emotion to be released, like anger or grief. Over time, we begin to have compassion for ourselves for feeling the emotion of fear.

Judgments get in the way of having what I want. For example, with regards to money, I could say: "I release the belief that I could never have as much money and prosperity as I want without working hard every day for forty years". Put another way, "I forgive myself for having believed for so long that the only way to have prosperity and/or a lot of money is to work for it". Parts of ourselves respond to such declarations.

These releases are about *undoing the spells* we've woven against ourselves. The difference can be noticed between these statements intending to release these judgments, and re-stating the judgment, such as "I just can't get enough money to satisfy my needs and desires!" That reiteration, as has been stated, magnetizes the situation to continue where I don't have enough.

Judgments Vs. Affirmations

Judgment release is different than making affirmations. Judgments are beliefs already present with us from bygone days. They are held in our energy field and shape our experience. We draw in or magnetize what we believe. The universe brings us what we believe will happen or is "supposed to" happen. Truth and pleasurable experiences cannot flow into the Self through a thick tangle of mental judgments, which redirect the universe to give us what we believe is real and true, even if it hurts us and even if we do not like it.

Affirmations, on the other hand are declarations of things that we have, do, or are that may or may not currently exist as a reality. The intent with affirmations is to obtain what we want or draw it by saying it's already the case. This is a different animal altogether from verbal judgment release.

Here are some examples of affirmations:

→I am wealthy beyond measure.

→I am healthy in all ways.

→I am happy and make others happy by being around them.

→My value is noticed and appreciated

Affirmations are of the spirit. They indicate eternal truths outside the bounds of space and time. While ideal and true if our potential was fully reached, affirmations do not necessarily reflect our present reality here in this body at this moment. Though some may try, affirmations cannot trump the denials and pain our emotional and mental bodies are holding that contradict the messages in the affirmation. They can be good triggers because they are so far from present reality, but are not effective tools for manifesting because of the inherent power within time and space of held emotional and mental energy.

Words are indeed spells, and if you do not believe me, examine your awareness sometime and write down all the judgments you hold about culture, reality and life, and see how much your manifestations and your emotional response to life and others or lack thereof is reflected by them. Judgments and beliefs about things and others were put into place in declared, verbal words, or thoughts, which have a certain power, i.e. a spoken spell. Releasing such beliefs out loud, or even clearly and formally but silently in your mind (I like both ways, just to be sure!) is a form of spell unmaking, creating magic that helps us get more of what we want and less of what we do not. This can be done by releasing old stagnant mental energy that prevents us from seeing experiences afresh for what they really are.

Acceptance

I no longer believe that I am anything outside of love
I no longer believe that it's bad to be
A tiny frightened dove
I am a window, the water and a wave
Sometimes an outlaw a jailor and a slave
I just want to be me, accept my right to just be

I no longer believe that I need do
What they say must be done

I no longer believe that there's a race
My fear says must be won
I am a window the water and a wave
Sometimes a hero a puppet a knave
I just want to be free, accept responsibility

My body my desire lead me ever higher
What was lost does now aspire
To be called home by the fire
Of our love

I no longer believe that we are anything outside of love
I no longer believe that it's bad
To be tiny frightened doves
We are the windows, the water and the waves
The hidden, healing saviours in our caves
We who want to be free must accept that reality

Chapter 18: Heal The Past to Change The Future

"Be here now." "Staying present." "Grounding into body." New age catch-phrases that can leave us thinking 'Yeah, sure, ok ...so how do we do this?' New-ageisms can sound too pat nowadays, and we want something more concrete, some applicable awareness that can help us heal our lives.

Try this one on for size – I am safe if I stay put in my current moment, breathing, doing, being...whatever I am doing and being. I cannot be hurt if I am in my body, fully. When I jump ahead of myself, when I spin future pictures based on assumptions, judgments and plans of various sorts, I am by definition "out of the moment" and generating fear, or excitement. It is either "going to be so bad" or "going to be so good".

When fear is generated by the passing pictures, the fear is not often processed. And this is how I set myself up for "reversals", i.e. experiences that set me back. By generating more fear that is not then processed, I put myself in danger, without even realizing it. Unprocessed fear and the judgments that accompany it have a tendency to attract the very experience feared. And of course, when I do feel afraid, it is vital to feel and organically express the fear, not technique or rationalize it away. Refrain from judging fear wrong or bad to exist. "I release the judgment that my fear is wrong to be."

How to return to the moment when you have left it to engage in future thoughts? When you realize it, you can withdraw immediately from the future, by choice. Just come back, accepting that you left for a while. You can cease to think about those future thoughts right now, feel your feet, the chair or floor beneath you, etc. and come back to your body and your moment. Look at what's right in front of you.

When The Moment For Decision Comes, The Choice Will Be Obvious.

My fear has been that if I allowed myself to stay completely present, letting the pictures of future possibilities roll by unexplored, that I would constantly get blindsided and be unprepared for incoming situations. Yet what does "prepared" really mean? Armed to the teeth with expectations of how I am going to handle the situation that has not yet come to pass? That behavior only locks the future into the past. I cannot allow magic, epiphany and serendipity into my new moments if I have already decided how I will respond and act ahead of time. When I do that, I miss the impact of the new experience and my organic response to it.

The tendency to want to do this reveals a mistrust of self. Mistrusting ourselves isn't wrong. It's okay to mistrust ourselves and recognize that mistrust is a reality until we organically come into trust over time. We need to have compassion for ourselves if we can't accomplish any or all of these steps outlined in the book right away.

If I do feel a need to nail down my future response ahead of time to a future situation, it can be helpful to notice without self-blame that I am in effect not trusting myself to be able to respond appropriately in the moment.

How will I make informed decisions without considering all the angles in advance? I can ask for inner guidance in the moment if I have time, and accept that I have the power to KNOW what to do when the right time comes for acting and responding. Taking full responsibility for my experiences, including my old imprints of victimization and perpetration, means accepting and getting comfortable with my ability to respond. My ability to respond not only means what feels like right, true, and often obvious action in the moment; it also means cultivating an ability to respond to my feelings with true depth of expression whenever I notice I am triggered. This means accepting where I had responsibility in a situation and letting myself and others know about this responsibility.

Response-ability in these areas generates acceptance. This acceptance affords a greater sense of comfort with myself, which leads to an increasing ease with staying present in my body. Over time, this growing ease manifests a sense of trust and safety in my world instead of more fear and danger.

The Past As Part of the Present

The past is where we were traumatized, and the past is what we are learning from. The past affects us, and guides us. Many judgments and unprocessed emotions from the past still affect everything happening in the present. To change the present, we must deal with the fallout from the past.

The NOW moment can expand to include sometimes necessary, even crucial explorations of the past. Our emotional processes can lead us down a track to explore the roots of our current trigger or judgment history. It is helpful and *necessary* to allow ourselves to follow our feeling bodies back into the past while staying rooted in our bodies, feeling the earth or floor beneath us while we engage in this.

Staying present, staying here, and therefore staying safe does not mean cutting off the past. Some songs and traditional spiritual or new age teachings encourage us to Be Here Now by pretending the past does not exist or no longer affects us since it's "gone". These teachings say the past does not continue to affect the present. Unfortunately, this input is steering us down a primrose path, which is attractive to some parts of us because it encourages us to dump out or cut off parts of ourselves trapped in the past. What is a primrose path, but a path that isn't real, a path of believing that that glossing over reality is doable? Denying how the past affects our present moment often seems easier. Denying can look like less work than working with past pain, but it does catch up with us and eventually brings the reversal of fortune we are trying to avoid.

The parts of me that are trapped in the past are parts that are holding unresolved emotions and judgments. Musing on past pictures can be a signpost that there is unresolved emotion there, or even entire parts of myself that I have split off and abandoned "back there". To redeem these parts of myself and bring them into the current moment, I need to enter whatever emotional door opens to me in the moment in which such daydreaming reveals one.

Staying present is not the same as blocking out all thoughts, it means naturally being able to focus and be "here and now" without trying very hard. If I am feeling at stasis emotionally, I can genuinely stay present.

Emotions are like time portals or pathways; they form lines back down the timeline to past realities and forward to future realities. We can reel ourselves in to the Now Moment from the past or future, becoming more safe and whole in the process by doing our work of healing and dealing.

Chapter 19: Asses Out of You and Me

"Well, I just assumed you knew." "You assumed I would not be up for it?" "I went on an assumption that we would never make it on time." Ahhhhhh, yes -- the assumption hole. We magically transform normal homo sapiens into braying donkeys, performing this dark, calcifying wizardry on ourselves and others on a daily basis (with due apologies to our full-time burro amigos).

How often have we uttered or heard word-for-word recitals of the above? How often does assuming we know what is real for a given moment match what is really happening? So often after our assumptions have proven faulty, we sheepishly grin to our partners or friends, "y'know, I was wrong about that thing" -- or we polarize and say something that defends the assumption, or the reasons for making the assumption.

Either way there are a few things I may have done there. First, I may have felt I had all the information I needed to 'safely' make an assumption. Secondly, I may have been operating on old information and failed to check back in to see if it was still true. Thirdly, I may have been running on fear. If so, this would have led to making the assumption. I may have fear of confronting the source of my fear. We may feel lack of safety around the source itself, be it a person or place or thing. I may have fear of admitting that I do not know everything already. I may have fear of success, which subconsciously sabotages a situation in order to prove judgments such as "nothing ever works" or "life sucks".

Hidden Fear Driving Assumptions

Healing the fear around knowing the truth could be a key to discovering why we make so many assumptions in our daily lives. Judgments about checking in or "bothering someone else" is one way this fear can manifest. Releasing such fears is crucial in order to regularly make decisions that work for us instead of backfiring.

Allowing and accepting fear's existence is the key to true release, including allowing it to move through you however it will. In a quiet moment, try touching into a fear of a situation, interaction, or person and see if you can contact root fears and judgments that lead to your assumptions about them/it. See if you can detect fear energy in your body. You can release fear through sound that wants to organically emerge directly from the energy you have contacted in your mind or body, through chattering teeth, shivering etc.

Perhaps the fear will leave you without you having to emotionally vibrate it, but do not just banish it. Ask what it needs and give it, including the right to move on. Acknowledging and/or expressing fear can release it; but banishing, or denying fear tends to split the parts of Self feeling the fear from the rest of the Self.

I said in the first paragraph of this chapter that internal "calcification", indicating mental, physical, and emotional stuckness, is part of the assumption process. Assumptions, close cousins of judgments, spring from stuck energy in my mind and emotions, which are reflected by the hard places in my physical musculature.

Assumptions reveal that I have chosen, perhaps unconsciously, not to try very hard to acquire all the information I can about a situation, person, place or thing. It sometimes may take more effort to acquire the information necessary to make a really educated choice or conclusion. Ani DiFranco said, "dig deeper, dig deeper this time" and that is what we assumers all need to do inside and outside ourselves if a more flowing and pleasant set of experiences is to befall us as a matter of course.

Death is Inevitable (And Other Judgments)

The following was written by Jean Gordy and is reprinted here by permission:

"What if I told you that death isn't inevitable. It seems like a ludicrous statement to make. When we look around us, clearly we can see by the evidence that everything dies eventually.

What if I told you that your consciousness is partly responsible for the death you see all around you, including your own death. What if I told you that if you want, you can turn the death imprint around, end the death cycle in your reality.

If that bit of information makes you angry, then good. Get mad, stomp your feet, yell and tell me that I am INSANE. You can even leave now if you want to; stop reading. Or you could suspend judgment for just a bit and keep reading and see if I have anything to say that might be worth sticking around for. Have I got your attention?

The belief in death is such a sacred cow. One of our favorite sayings is 'nothing in life is for sure except death and taxes.' Earth is an interesting place. When we look around, we see such a homogenized reality. It seems we are 'fed' our reality by 'The System'. We are told how to live by 'The Experts'. We are told what the median life span for the human being is. We go to a doctor to find out what is wrong with our bodies, and what we need to do to heal them. We are told if we can recover from a serious illness, and even told how long we will live if something like cancer is found in our bodies.

Can you imagine how being told something such as when we are going to die by an outside authority must affect us? And the results are mixed. Some people rally around and say 'screw that' and go on living, maybe even actually healing themselves. Others just lay down and die.

Certainly, living a stressful life, or doing something in life that we hate doing has an effect on how fast we age. Imagine how a life that was lovely, pleasant, beautiful, fulfilling and stress-free would affect our health and our longevity. But certainly, even if we had all the things in life that supported a long life, certainly we would eventually die anyway. Or would we? How do we even know if we've never had the chance to experience a pleasant and stress-free life?

Then that brings up the immediate problem of the difficulties we run into just trying to survive on the planet at this time. It seems most people are stressed to the   max. Some die young, some get some debilitating disease and spend most of their lives struggling to live, some live to a ripe old age. If you look around, it looks like a crap shoot to me.

So the idea of turning around this imprint around death, or even just being able to extend our lives in a fulfilling way seems to need our attention before we can even contemplate the possibility that not dying is even an option.

So let's start there. It seems that the world is getting harder and harder to survive in. We use our intelligence to look around us and many of us find life getting denser, harder and requiring more struggle than ever to survive. Why is this so? Are we just victims to the reality around us? It sure feels so sometimes. I was raised in an environment of struggle. My parents were almost always struggling for money. My personal imprint is lack, so lack in my life is a personal theme. Over the years it has become apparent to me that at a deep level, I believe that life is hard, that I have to work hard in order to survive. I look around at others who seem to draw in what they need so easily. This has made me very angry at times, but I have also seen that I am not very comfortable with prosperity. I don't trust it. And I have an imprint that if it comes, it's just going to be a matter of time before it goes. And waiting for that shoe to drop can be darn scary.

So how does all this relate back to the death imprint? Through my own personal imprinting I have created for myself a stressful life that has created ongoing illness for me that I have had to spend a lot of time addressing and plumbing deeply to find the root causes of. Through my years of investigation, and a very strong personal imperative to 'keep living', I have sought out solutions and understandings for myself. I have done the work to heal the difficulties that I have manifested in my life. And I say I have manifested these because I take responsibility for all that I have manifested. It is mine to heal. I've also had lots of help from significant information that I have rooted out from research, and from surrounding myself with like-minded people that are on the same questing path that I am.

So even though I am not fully healed, even though I am still aging, I have found solutions to many of my problems and issues, and slowly but surely, I am turning my life around."

Chapter 20: Honestly!

What is truth? Truth is our subjectively honest input, subject to change with more information and experience. What is "our truth in the moment"? Our truth can be found in what we perceive, what we do, say, feel, believe or think. We have been told as children to "tell the truth, now". We have taken in many messages since that time that revealing "the truth, the whole truth, and nothing but the truth" is what shapes our character and integrity. I resonate with this to a large extent, while also knowing that honesty and truth-telling is fraught with old pain and damage for many of us.

In all likelihood, it is necessary over time to release judgments about a person, place, thing or situation first in order to know our truth more fully and clearly. Only then can we be centered in our truth.

We have trauma around revealing truth and not being believed. We have trauma around being punished for revealing truth, an indicator that guilt is present. When we have given all we have to give and are met with mistrust and suspicion, it is a grave indicator that we contain large gaps of mistrust of ourselves being reflected by the person facing us. We have trauma around feeling too afraid to reveal key parts of the truth. This unprocessed fear and denied guilt generates its worst nightmare when somehow the withheld information is discovered and the other person responds with feelings of betrayal and hurt. Additionally, we have trauma around the guilt we feel when our truth triggers someone else into their hurt.

This guilt within can look like punishment from without. On the personal scale we have been punished for lying, telling partial truths, and for telling the whole truth. On the global scale, withholding or even revealing the truth has resulted in torture, death or perpetration of crimes against humanity.

The Hiding-Spilling Continuum

The consequence of these seminal scenes in our pasts around giving our truth is that our behaviour can warp when faced with another opportunity to speak our truth to another. Perhaps we find ourselves situated somewhere near one pole of the hiding/spilling continuum. On one end, we are mostly or completely withholding our truths. On the other we reveal every low-level detail we can think of regardless of its appropriateness to the situation at hand. Neither polarity offers a balanced response. Releasing fear and judgments, then bringing in compassion, with true heart present, is the only way the truth is real as truth, and the only way it can be easily received.

Sometimes we are more prone to hide information. This can stem from shame that we have done something wrong, or have been "bad". We hide information when we fear repercussions, or judge that certain reactions are inevitable if we share. We fear or judge that we may hurt others with our truth, or lose their love. Chronic hiding from others may indicate that we chronically hide truth and awareness from ourselves as a matter of course. We can fear that revealing truth will "say something" about us that isn't going to feel good. When we hide, we are often allowing these fears or judgments to act out. Chronic hiding also creates a mild but noticeable "criminal" energy in our field and results in people not trusting us or feeling fully relaxed, spontaneous and genuine around us.

Conversely there are times when revealing an entirety of truth may well endanger us. At these times, we must trust our wills to tell the truth as we see fit, tailored to our audience. There is no formula here, and each situation must be felt in the moment.

Without emotional movement in this arena, the pendulum may easily swing to the "spilling" end of the continuum, where we reveal every little detail, sometimes above and beyond. Imagine revealing a past crime to a police officer who has pulled you over for a traffic violation, because you couldn't hold back the need to spill.

This is of course an extreme example. The compulsion to spill or the action taken to spill minutia of detail is often resulting from guilt. We spill to relieve ourselves of as much guilt as possible. Sometimes spilling is necessary and integral to a situation. Speaking slowly can help us to catch up with whether we are revealing appropriately in a given situation.

When we withhold the truth or communicate an outright lie, we set up a split inside ourselves, where one side holds the known truth, willfully hidden from the other, while another part of ourselves speaks the lie. Recalling that words are spells that can work for or against us, setting up this split engenders a harmful magic, ultimately against ourselves.

Emotional and spiritual process can be vital ahead of time in order to get clear on where to land within the hiding/spilling continuum. Engaging in this process helps to more accurately align with our own inner sense of what feels right to reveal as opposed to "what we should say". Judgments such as "they cannot handle the truth" are distorted evaluations predicated on past pain and experience. Before approaching someone with a potentially sensitive truth, we may have some work to do first. Releasing any judgments, predictions and projections out loud ahead of time if possible around what to say and how much or little is right to say can be extremely helpful.

Truth Begets Trust

The payoff of finding a balanced truth to give in each situation is the growth of trust: trust for self, trust for other, and trust for the truth itself. The cultivation of trust is most important in long-term relationships, where investing my deepest truth in each moment becomes paramount. When I am in the midst of speaking the real truth, there is a sense of ease, love, trust, and compassion.

How do I get there? Expressing emotions and judgments ahead of time in the ways described in this book can be very helpful. Noticing my intuitive sense of just what to say and how to say it, perhaps after an expression session is a huge key. Intuition often presents as my "still, small voice" that has a different qualitative feel to it than mentally grinding out a solution amidst the din and clatter of unexpressed charge. Daring to notice and follow my intuitive guidance can result from intention to pay attention to my deeper Knowing and cultivation of the art of inner listening. Learning how to "think on my feet" in the midst of an interaction where I am revealing information is a part of the art of truth telling. If "blanking out' is a repeating pattern in these situations where thinking on one's feet would have helped, you can be sure that there is hidden emotion beneath the blankness. You can always go back and address this later, especially if a truth reveal did not go well.

Let's look at some classic judgments around truth telling. As described in Chapter 2 of this section, there are several forms of judgment release that can be applied, which I randomly give examples of in the following judgment possibilities. Out loud in a safe space, give as much emotional weight as you can to each of the following releases that apply to your particular belief system:

→ "I release the judgment that (person x) can't handle the truth.

→ "I release the judgment that it is not safe for me to tell my truth to most people.

→ "I forgive myself for having believed for so long that if I hold back in any way, it will be found out eventually.

→ "I release the judgment that telling every bit of the truth that I can find keeps me safe.

→ "I release the judgment that I can't hide things from myself.

→ "I intend to release the belief that I am not capable of revealing truth in a balanced way in each and every situation.

→ "I release the judgment that giving the whole truth is brutal honesty and is therefore unloving.

→ "I reject the belief that certain truths land in people like being punched in the gut, and that that is all my responsibility."

Any others that come to mind from engaging in this exercise can be considered appropriate releases if they occur to you.

Without knowing how to give my truth, I cannot develop the trust I need in myself or in anybody else. Being in my deepest truth can grow with practice, becoming more facile with time and deeds. Being in my truth keeps me safe, because when I speak truth I am in harmony with as much of myself as I possibly can be in the moment. When I can be true to myself first and foremost, thoroughly honest with myself at all levels, it can radiate outward into all of my relationships.

Chapter 21: Extreme Self-Love

{This chapter was written by Bee Wolf-Ray (http://earthmatrix.net) and reprinted here with permission.}

The Secret, and similar programs all involve changing the shape of thoughts through the exercise of will; in other words, thinking differently in order to harness the power of positive thoughts to create a better reality for ourselves. Considerations of what sort of reality we try to create with these thoughts aside, it is a very good idea, but like many good ideas, there are problems in practice.

In my experience, darker thoughts often spontaneously rise to contradict conscious intent, and this effectively cancels out positive reality-creation potential. Part of me believes while another part sneers in the background, seeing only the shadow cast by the light.

Example: "I love myself. I am beautiful," evokes an immediate, hidden, unconscious response: "What a crock. Nobody else loves me. I am ugly even if I think I am beautiful." I can say positively, "Cancel that thought," or "I release the judgment that nobody loves me and I am ugly," which helps, but until I get at the root causes for these thoughts, changes are merely cosmetic.

Becoming aware of the echoes and unconscious reactions to attempts to change and grow is an enlightening process, though changing the pattern of the thoughts is not quite as simple and easy as choosing differently, regardless of what 'they say'.

In my experience and understanding, such rebellious and reactive thoughts simply cannot be controlled, and when we attempt to exert control, we fan the flames of our internal war which is reflected by the external conflicts plaguing the planet. Peace begins within, and is not attained by pouring oil on troubled waters nor through any form of enforced discipline. This is a consensus reality, and until we achieve true (i.e., unforced) inner consensus, the majority will rule: so far, the majority of our being is confined to the subconscious.

These parts of self know something that the conscious mind does not, and yes, they are sullen, rebellious, angry and intractable. Why shouldn't they be? They know exactly how little we trust them, how unwilling we really are to face them, ask them who they are and what they really want. They know us better than we know them, for the divers in the deep can clearly see the swimmers in the light who circle above them, but the light-centric selves are blind to the denizens of the darkness, not to mention uninterested and judgmental.

When we judge some thoughts to be good and others to be bad, rather than exploring all thoughts from source to consequence, we ignore and effectively deny our power. The negative matters, yes, and we do know its potential for destructiveness; that is why we are so earnestly bent on controlling it. But we have no idea what might happen if we truly embrace our negativity and ask it to teach us what it knows.

Thought experiment:

Positive thought: "I am radiant and creative." Negative response: "I am so full of shit."

Ask: who said that?
Answer: somebody who knows your secrets.
Ask: what secrets?
Answer: everything, and I mean everything that you do
not like is within you. There is no escape from your
shadow.

Solution seems obvious: embrace and love what
you have not liked. Sounds simple, but it is not easy to
pull off. We need to humble ourselves in the face of our
dark, angry, hurting, frightened, cynical selves, to accept
that just maybe they know something we do not. We have
(the conscious ego) sought knowledge for so long, and
attempted to teach, train, condition and control our
subconscious minds which seem the source of so much
unruliness, chaos and anxiety, but never have we slowed
our search down and simply asked our wayward feelings,
what do you know that I do not know?

Answer: everything.
Ask: such as?
Answer: the premises of the reality under which you
operate are fundamentally flawed. Erase and start over.

We do not like to hear that answer, nor do we
want to believe it. Still, to pretend it is wrong just because
it is inconvenient to believe appears insanely self-
destructive. According to the view from below where such
things can be seen, the very foundations of reality are
cracked and rotten. All attempts to heal it have so far
taken the form of concealing the rot, not changing
anything in any real way. It is like painting over rotting
floorboards and covering them with a nice carpet, then
acting surprised when the floor caves in.

Somewhere in the basement an alarm bell is
clanging and all the positive thinking, profound discipline
and learning in Creation will not make it stop. Only

stopping what we are doing and letting ourselves feel how scared and angry we really are will do that, or at least open space to feel what to do and where to go next.

When we stop, we can feel the movement of the spheres, we can hear ourselves breathing. When we end the constant stream of mental lectures and instructions directed toward our lesser selves, we can begin to hear their point of view.

Body knows things that Mind does not. The flow of understanding has to start to move in different grooves, through circulating loops of feedback, and the knowledge cannot source from somebody else's system, not ever. We have to feel our way through the particular weaving winding multidimensional labyrinth that is our own personal path, and nobody can teach us how.

Our body is our guide and guru, and it is only mind's egotistical pride that insists on resisting the impulses that come from our physical wisdom. Body is always right, even when it is wrong. Indulging in your compulsions is the only way to understand them, but you have to do it with attention and intention to understand, not throwing up mind's hands and surrendering in a huff, saying, "Ok, you get your way, wake me when you need me for inevitable damage control."

Our body needs the rest of ourselves to stay awake and alive no matter what, no matter how it looks or feels, and to seek the self-trust that provides the magic ingredient for alchemizing our experience.

We learn by doing; we will know we are there only when we actually are there. We will be healed of addictions when we no longer crave them, but the path of resistance can never take us to that desired end. We will always desire things that our mind judges to be wrong until our mind stops judging and starts seeking to understand the meaning of what happens while it is happening.

Our mind is blind, deaf and dumb, the victim of the numbing barrage from the collective mental freak-out, the rebellious, reactive shouting of the unconscious masses. We need to stop listening to them, and start listening to our Selves.

When craving with blind raging desire to stuff yourself with sweetness, oblivion or altered awareness, do not fight the craving. Give in consciously and stay self-lovingly aware as you indulge. Taste what you eat, notice how you feel while in altered states, breathe into your experience with curiosity and the will to accept and understand. Break habits of thought and control first, and physical habits will follow when they are really ready. Do not say grudgingly to yourself, "Alright, but just this once." Do not impose conditions or condescend.

Give in lovingly, compassionately, without superior understanding. Know that you do not know what it means, and accept not knowing. Seek not answers from books, teachers or anyone outside your own body of truth. Ask the Consciousness of the Whole for help and support in your journey.

Forgive yourself. Constantly. Forgive yourself, not for what you do, but for the ways that you judge what you do to be bad, wrong, unhealthy or otherwise unacceptable in your own eyes. Forgive your own conditional love for your sweet self. Forgive your petty criticisms, your assumptions and your arrogance. Accept all of your being, the light and the dark, and listen to all of your thoughts, the positive and the negative. Negative thoughts have a teaching to offer: they let you know that a part of you is unhappy with what you are thinking or doing. This does not mean, cave in blindly to every unhappy voice. It means, give each unhappy voice your loving attention and allow its response to be your own. Own it, in other words, as yourself.

Sample situation: suppose you are at a meditation retreat for the purpose of raising your vibration and becoming a more positive and fulfilled being. You are chanting mantras and doing breathing exercises in a group.

You are aware of an unhappy voice in the background of your mind:

"This is bullshit. I hate this."
Query from consciousness: "What do you hate about it?"
"It is stupid and annoying."
"What is stupid about it?"
"Nobody asked me how I felt about doing this. I hate sitting still. I hate repeating rote thoughts as formulas."
"What can I do, seeing as how we are here and committed to the experience, to make it better for you?"
"Listen to me. Feel me."

Then, allow yourself to do it. Feel how much you hate what you are doing, without abandoning your awareness of the other parts of yourself which are enjoying and thriving in the experience. It is you thinking these things, after all. These thoughts tell a truth about how you really feel that you have not noticed because you believed that to feel it would interfere with having a good experience. Allow the goodness to continue and embrace the badness at the same time. You can do it. You are a great being with room for many internal contradictions and a wide variety of experience. Do not ignore your sad hurting selves.

If a baby cries at a party, somebody needs to care for it, yet the party can go on. Your unhappy thoughts are your own babies crying. You are responsible to them, and ignoring them has long-term consequences.

Allow your body to shift in small ways, to shiver, to quiver in indignation at imposed stillness. Inasmuch as you feel safe to do so, allow small sounds. Notice

149

everything about how it feels to be doing this, stretch your awareness to its limit. Exercise your loving attention. Let your attention go toward, not stopping or controlling your negativity, but increasing and expanding your awareness, acceptance and understanding of yourself. Keep yourself safe by allowing your expression to be appropriate in the context of the situation, and love all parts of you.

Be lovingly-intended toward yourself. You deserve it. All of you.

* * * * * * * *

Part IV

The Spiritual Body

Chapter 22: The Embodied Spirit

There are many beliefs and confusions about what spirit is. Some believe we are nothing but spirit if we were to be rendered down into our basic aspects. Others say we need to escape the earthly shell of our bodies and arrive at a spiritual destination. Still others believe there is no such thing as a personal spirit.

Our spiritual body comprises one of the four parts of the divinity we each embody. Our spirit gives us an overview of any situation we are involved in. Spirit sees all the options of a situation. Our desire body, also known as the emotional body or will, then makes a free choice about which option to engage in. If our body is willing to try it and our heart is in it, we step into action.

Our spirit guides us. At opportune times, often after emotional movement and process has occurred, spirit witnesses the overview of a situation. Spirit can then offer prospective solutions or possibilities that could help us evolve and move toward what would feel good to us in the short or long run. Spirit also helps us name what we are going through, brings us clarity of thought connected to the emotional experience. Without Spirit's help, the emotional self feels lost in dreamlike chaos.

The Resistance To Embodiment Within Spirit

There are those who would say that embodying the whole Self is not something worthwhile and that spirit is the be-all and end-all of existence. Such a point of view might be expressed thusly: "Are you suggesting I not be in the Oneness all the time? You can't be saying you want me to go and experience *that*? That's far too messy for me. Emotions flaring up at a moment's notice? Body pain? No thank you. I'll just be here, meditating on the light. Why should I have to go where they are? They can come up here and be with me if they want me! Soooooo unevolved, that 'basic self'."

In certain pockets of the so-called New Age movement, even hinting that the spiritual body of a person is not already perfect and exalted beyond the need for evolution is tantamount to blasphemy. After all, aren't our spirits perfect reflections of the perfect God, who "obviously" has no need to evolve? One thing necessary for mind and spirit to notice, however, is that the prevailing attitude inherent in the monologue above has not achieved healing on the planet to date. In fact, it may be important for this part of our being to notice that we seem to be heading in the opposite direction of healing as a species en toto.

The "rise above it" philosophy is not the answer. Perhaps true Oneness is not just Oneness of that which is already Light, but Oneness of all essence, which is in fact comprised of the physical, emotional, mental and spiritual.

In the secular world, the attitude betrayed by scientists is that spirit cannot be proven, therefore it does not exist. It does not matter to scientific folks if we have subjective experiences of our own spirit, when science's instruments cannot measure its length and breadth.

A Body In Pain's Need For Spirit

It behooves all parts of our being, especially the spiritual body, to descend fully into the physical and come to balance with all parts of the self, if human beings are to achieve healing as connected individuals and as a whole. A hugely important key to healing everything in us is full commitment of our spiritual selves (or *consciousness*) to stay present and embodied. Spirit needs to be a participating and responsive part of the self's healing. A detached Spirit "observing" Body's situation from above by definition is split apart from Body and does not allow for healing. Body requires Spirit to be within in order to truly exist in its fullest healing potential. Conversely, Spirit requires Body in order to be manifest on Earth.

The next time you are in pain, allow yourself, with intent to do so and willingness to drop distractions, to become fully present at the heart of that pain, be it emotional or physical. Drop as deeply into the center of your pain as you can, and stay there for as long as you can, feeling and experiencing all that you feel and experience. Instead of rising above the pain, allow your consciousness to sink into it. Breathing into the center of the pain is a form of acceptance that can shift the pain...part of pain's persistence is our resistance to it, our attempt to quell or push it away or twist away from it. Usually pain has some sort of message, even if indirect and non-obvious.

You will know you are successful if you experience a qualitative shift from "pain" to "sensation". Twisting away from the center of the pain makes it hurt even more and causes us to engage the habitual cycle of reaching for the nearest avenue of pain relief. Pain is a message from Body. Twisting away from the pain is a form of habituated avoidance of this message.

Meditation on Your Pain

Here is a meditation on dealing with pain. You can have someone read this to you or recite it into a recording unit to play back to yourself while you sit comfortably.

Close your eyes and deeply breathe into the center of the pain, feeling all of what you experience, emotionally or physically. Go to the heart of the pain with your awareness – let go now of all outside distraction and sit in the center of it as much as you consciously can. Imagine that you are a deep-sea diver entering a cave, breathing light into the strong feelings or physical sensations of pain as you cry them, moan them, scream them, gasp, choke, tremble, allow the half dead sounds or simply quietly feel them. Pay attention to the feelings and the expression from your emotions, let yourself sink in and be aware, present, noticing everything.

Just sit in this space. If doing so does not shift the pain, ask it its message, out loud, as sound vibration matters to our physical bodies - what does it want from me, what does it want me to know? Let your parts in pain know that you are receiving and accepting this message now. Feel into the shape of the pain, its color and texture. Ask it if it's a part of you trying to come home. Usually pain wants us to feel something we've been avoiding. Where in me, in my field or body, does it belong? What part of me is it? If I have been avoiding this essence, or if I have unknowingly caused this part of me pain by previously going past my limits or done something to hurt myself out of my ignorance, I can apologize to it for that, and see what doing so brings up.

Medication

None of us like pain, it can be extremely difficult to deal with and we have been trained from a very young age to use strong medicine to quell its symptoms and message. Many people habitually reach for pain medication immediately upon awareness of pain. This is not wrong per se, but it blocks off consciousness. Minimize pain medication to the point where you only take it if you feel you must have it.

Notice how your experience shifts when your spiritual body drops in. Accept what is going on without trying to channel or suppress it in any way. Breathe deeply, slowly, and without effort or push, if that is possible. Doing so is more than a meditation, it is pure experience, even if it's only seconds at a time before you jump out. The spirit has tremendous power to effect healing with its mere presence, co-existing fully in physical experience with the rest of you in a completely present moment. Receiving all that you feel without judgment can bring huge shifts. If necessary, release judgments as described in Part 3. The longer and more often you can practice full conscious presence in your pain, the better, faster and more effective your healing the issue at hand can be.

Do Not "Go" To Heaven – Bring It Here!

There is a common belief in New Age, in Buddhism, in Christianity, in Islam, that the body is something to be shed like a shell, because the goal is to get to heaven with just your spirit. My problem with that is, when there is only Spirit present, the rest of the Self is absent. Spirit alone cannot substitute for the whole person.

My vision is that we move towards co-creating heaven on Earth, where we all have bodies of light, with passion and senses intact, with all magic and powers present without giving anything up to do so. To get to that place we need *all* parts of ourselves to be fully functional and present and not just our spirits. The end of death and dying must happen for this to manifest. That is what I want, not some spiritual way-station between mixed-bag lives of struggle and fleeting moments of joy between long jags of torpor, misery and dullness.

"Jesus said, 'You have been given eternal life in your own name. When you are able to comprehend the grandeur of that gift, you will be able to experience your birth anew with ecstasy.'"[1]

I would add, "and when you are able to release all of the emotional pain and imprinting you took in from your original experiences and misconceptions that you have held and denied ever since the beginning, your gaps and splits within will close and heal and you will be reborn in ecstasy".

[1] *Glenda Green, "Love Without End – Jesus Speaks", chapter 3*

Chapter 23: Not So Hasty

Many of us are familiar with the character Treebeard from Tolkien's "Lord Of The Rings" and the comical ways in which he moved and acted more slowly than any of the other characters (who were not Ents, of course). We could say that nobody in a human body would ever want to take as long as Treebeard did to do things, but I find Treebeard to be a great teacher. When I am moving slowly and unhurriedly, my breathing deepens, my thoughts drop out, I feel my spirit integrating more deeply into my body and I am significantly more in touch with my body and my feelings. Remembering and practicing the art of slowness is tricky to master.

Those of us blessed to live in rural settings figure we have slowed down the pace of our lives merely by living there, having "dropped out of the race". To some extent this is true, but we need only look to how we behave during tourist season, or any time of year where busy-ness increases, to notice how extremely we pressure ourselves to pick up the pace. Though we can strive to, and some of us succeed in living mostly off the grid, we cannot separate from the rest of our species. The world is getting faster, and from inside ourselves we feel impelled to keep up. Television, and especially commercials, faster than ever in their jump cuts, are a reflection of this. Notice how Facebook and other social media makes us reach for "fast food" information/distractions, and also how frustrated we become when the limitations of the computer slow down our habitual internet usage.

Fear of Death

There are many possible reasons for this phenomenon, but one stands out: fear of death. This fear could be described as a fear of not getting everything we want done before we start to become decrepit and become incapable of realizing our dreams and doing everything we judge we need to do so that those dreams may reach fruition.

To compensate for this unresolved terror, we move fast. We get ahead of ourselves, we leave the moment and our bodies. We over-plan, strategize and scheme, our lightning-quick minds three moves ahead of whatever we are doing. We do not notice what our bodies are actually doing and feeling. We breathe shallowly and unconsciously. And from Middle Earth, Treebeard sighs and shrugs his shoulders.

Options for Slowing Down

What can be done to slow down and live deliberately? There are several possibilities to play with. Try taking some time every day to sit and breathe deeply and slowly for a few minutes. Then, while continuing to breathe, continue moving through your day in slow motion. It does not have to be ultra-slo-mo, just slower than your normal pace.

Notice what comes up in you as a result; do you feel impatience, harsh words in your head to "get a move on", with dire predictions of missed deadlines? That internal pressure to move faster is real; you are not making it up.

If you feel emotions arise as a result, allow them to express. This release process may look like expressing fear in sound that you won't fulfill your responsibilities, or rage that there just isn't enough time in the day – or it may be generalized frustration or fear – remember that you don't have to know what it's about before you release, and you don't have to justify the feelings "worthy" of expressing them. Expression is the key.

Personally, the best way I have found to cool down my own pace is a daily practice of Somatics exercises. They are a brilliant body meditation, an organic slowdown for my entire system, and contain a plethora of health benefits (see Part 1, Chapter 6 for more information on the practice of Somatics). I like to practice mindful movement when I have completed my daily routine. Yoga may accomplish the same things for you. It is important to find a body-centered practice that works for you if you intend to bring yourself present and reduce your "hastiness quotient".

We do sometimes need to move quickly in order to accomplish things in certain time frames. Of course, it is okay to move fast when you need to; this is not meant to make anyone feel guilty or wrong for moving expediently when necessary. Even Treebeard knows there is a time for action. Hom-hooooooom!!

Chapter 24: The Three Mo's

Remember the classic slapstick comedy team The Three Stooges: Moe, Larry and Curly? In the realms of personal change, there also exists another classic three, The Three Mo's: Motivation, Movement, and Momentum. These highly important, synergistic energies are keys for either proactively or reactively engendering advances on our personal evolutionary journey.

What do I mean by "proactively or reactively engendering advances"? Proactively engendering our personal evolution comes from taking proactive (from within oneself), intentional steps toward increasing or gathering momentum. One example of motivation in action, or movement to shift one's body toward greater health and joie de vivre is taking a supporting class in order to further excite one's Self (i.e. generate momentum) toward attaining the goal. Increased flexibility, more robust health, zest for life, and clearance of old pain are a few examples illustrating a class's intent that aligns with a desire we have to help our body shift. If we've chosen the right class for our needs, we experience movement that happens both within and outside the class environment toward our goal of greater health and well-being. Ongoing physical attendance at class, on a journey to realizing a personal desire can in even a short time spark further motivation.

Groups vs. DIY

Classes are not the only way to do this, for all one has to do is want a thing or state badly enough to "stoke the mo's" all on one's lonesome. Still, agreeing to meet where human energies are likewise engaged -- and this could be a 1-1 meeting, though classes carry greater collective energy and therefore greater momentum-building in potential -- can stimulate the latent seed of motivation perhaps languishing in judgments, inertia or hopelessness. Such a gathering could be a group of like-minded souls together in a room who happen to discuss a common desire and/or goals. Formality is not a pre-requisite to the ability of an intentional group to generate The Three Mo's.

Reactively engendering advances on our personal path of change most often comes in the form of healing from an injury or disease. We find motivation in the desire to survive or be as fully functional as possible again, particularly if we are faced with something life-threatening. Sometimes motivation can be encumbered by a lack of emotional movement. Old stagnant emotions, perhaps stirred by our situation, can stifle motivation, suppress movement and prevent momentum from being generated. There are stages of an illness, chronic pain or injury where we can feel overwhelmed into inaction by feelings of hopelessness, fatalism and repeating judgment loops on the theme of our "lot in life" in some way.

The Positive Feedback Loop

Motivational energy (aka desire) builds in the emotional body. Movement within can occur before outer movement. One flavor of movement is emotional expression. Old emotions are often "sitting" on our true desire to improve our energy and health. These emotions literally require movement before they can reach a state where they are working for the Self instead of against it. Once they "move" or express and have their say, motivation/desire can ideally be freed to stimulate right action and ultimately generate the all-important momentum, or directionality that creates the feedback loop back into increasing motivation, movement and momentum.

Once sufficiently underway, the feedback loop of motivation, movement and momentum proceeds on its own. The progression seems to "begin" from inward movement leading to motivation, then to outward movement or right action and then to momentum which then again feeds back into motivation and so on. With the Three Mo's activated, we are building the magic that leads to goal attainment and a quantum step along the healing path on the road to life and love and light.

Chapter 25: *Desiring Spirit and Cultivating Faith*

I talked about how spirit has to commit to the rest of the Self - the mental, emotional and physical bodies - in order for us as whole beings to be fully embodied and present. So what is our side of it, how do we have responsibility to draw our spirits to us, and keep them with us?

Desire Matters

Desire is a key. We call on the angels, we call on ascended masters, we call on devas, faeries and guides, we call on Jesus, we call on Buddha, we pray to God. The step we may have been missing here is to consciously call on our personal spirits to be present with us, to guide us, to help us be big, to bridge the gap to the Divine.

Our spiritual power is relatively untapped, and having a close, honest look at our misfired lives reveals a reflection of this latency, manifested as a lack of flow, a lack of abundance, a lack of grace. Certainly we all have moments and seasons of time when these gifts are present with us, but those moments pass, and quite often we find ourselves feeling as though having fallen from a great height, desiring, yet experiencing lack.

Certain bodies of so-called spiritual wisdom have wanted to distract us from our subjective reality's truth that we do indeed feel lack. We are told to look at all we have, look at how much better we have it than the people in (fill in name of third world country here). We have to get real with how we feel, and not compare ourselves out of our true feelings.

Achieving this balance can be complex. True, unadulterated desire for spirit can help draw and keep spirit present, but in our emotional bodies we have to deal with the hopelessness and old denied rages and hurts at having deeply desired spirit in the past only to have spirit not come no matter how much we wanted it to come. Some of us have judgments holding these old feelings in place that say, among other things, that desire for spirit's power is wrong, that desire to be one with our spirits does not help anyway so why bother feeling desire.

These judgments, and others like them, need release in the manner described in Part III ("The Mental Body"), as do the old, held feelings with them. The more we can do this, the more present our spirit can be with us, if we can dare to reach for it again. The more consciously magnetic we can become from vibrating our emotional bodies' huge magnetic storehouse and bringing it to life via expressing whatever is there to be expressed, the more we can literally attract and keep present our spirit, which is electric in its nature.

Our responsibility is that many of us have turned away from Spirit. We have judged that it is not possible to have a direct relationship with Spirit. I feel it is important in our personal evolution and our journey back to balance with the Divine to speak directly to Spirit, out loud, expect and listen for a response, and work through our blocks to trusting what we receive. Why out loud? Vibration matters, and sound is vibration. We need to let Spirit know our intentions, what we like and don't like, what kind of world we want to live in, and ask for the help we need in whatever forms we are capable of receiving that help. In this way we can initiate and reactivate our connection, and take responsibility for ourselves. In return, we can receive light and guidance that we can get nowhere else in the same way.

Expressing Emotions Magnetizes Spirit

Emotional expression is also a key in drawing and keeping spirit with us. The spirit is electric, the will or emotional body is magnetic, and when our magnetic self is vibrating, the law of electromagnetism is engaged and more of our loving light, our spirit self, is drawn to us to stay, not merely to make an appearance during a meditation only to float off again because we don't have any magnetic presence or much vibrating in that part of ourselves.

Healing for this part of us might look like asking Great Spirit, or God, or whatever our name for the Divine is to help guide our personal spirit back to us, to help our spirit integrate itself as part of the whole being, to help each of us know individually how to attract and keep our spiritual body present and aligned with us.

One last key aspect of healing with our spiritual bodies is cultivating a sense of faith that what we want, finding our right place and path in life, will come to us via our spirit once we call for our spirit's presence and begin to elevate the vibratory level of our emotional body. Trust and faith in whatever we call God, and in our spirit, can come once we move through all old anger and hopelessness and hurt towards Spirit for not being there for us in the past.

Dare To Burn

Dare to want that love,
Dare to want what's real
Dare to trust the wish to heal,
To want how it could feel
Dare to burn, dare to burn

Desire is a fire, a magnet pulling strong
We've been told in many ways that feeling it is wrong
Yet when I quell its flames, it brings a harvest anyway
Of many things I've feared,
And all the ashen shades of gray
When I don't dare to yearn, or dare to burn

Dare to want that gold, dare to want what's mine
Dare to trust that shiver that's travelling up my spine
Dare to burn

'Be careful what you ask for',
The ancient wisdom sings
But asking for and wanting
Are completely different things
To trust the wish to want the dream
The shining artist cast
Brings the moment that feels good
And the future to the past
When we dare to yearn, dare to burn

Saying and feeling are two different things
The words wisp away on some frail angel's wings
It can't float, it won't fly, it don't fall from the sky
Got to burn it here on the ground,
Get it moving, moving in sound
And groove with the rhythm it pounds,
To face up that ancient taunt that says,
"So…how does it feel to want??!!!"

Dare to want to live, dare to claim that space

Dare to buy the story that we're the saving grace
Dare to want that power, dare to pay that price
Dare to want the whole damn thing,
And not some random slice

Dare to want that love,
Dare to want what's real
Dare to trust the wish to heal,
To want how it could feel
Dare to burn, dare to burn

Prayer and Desire

There is a synergistic relationship between desire and prayer that is underplayed or outright omitted in the New Age and other religious literature. Praying with desire is how a close friend was able to draw a visceral, tangible presence of the Divine into her life.

One night she stood in the moonlight fervently praying for Spirit to enter her everyday life as a tangible presence. Burning with a radiating desire, she put out a direct call – 'be with me in a way I can feel and sense.' Spirit came immediately, letting her know she was experienced by the Divine as a bright attractive light that easily allowed her to be found.

In the days that followed, she felt Spirit right there with her in the room, a palpable presence she could as easily dialogue with as if you or I were sitting next to her in the room. She described it as going from a feeling of a "telephone hookup" (in her previous connections to the Divine) to a friend sitting beside her. As a result, she experienced a fulfillment and happiness she had never felt.

I believe she is able to have such a visceral experience of Spirit now because she burned her desire so fiercely that night. Our sensory experience of the Divine, and the manifestation wished for is going to be greater or more easily fulfilled if the element of desire is consciously allowed into the prayer itself.

Desire Cards

Here is another example from my own life. Several years ago, I read something on the internet that inspired me. I made a bunch of little cards that had desires written on them. Every day I drew one or more cards, like some people draw angel cards or medicine cards. If, at that moment, I felt as though I could still feel that desire in me that was on the card, I closed my eyes and let the desire upwell within me, reaching a state of meditative centeredness, maybe even feeling triggered by the feeling of need or want there.

Many of my desire cards were focused around abundance and manifestation in my life. After four straight months of giving relatively few massages, I wanted more opportunity to do my work and create some financial flow. I did this desire process in October, and then the following two months, November-December, were my two biggest months of the year. December's total massages were double October's. The subsequent Jan-Feb totals far exceeded previous years' Jan-Feb totals.

I had been simply praying and asking for abundance, without bothering to feel my desire or consciously allowing it to upwell within me, up until that point. Feeling how much I desire something is the key; one can't presume that the act of asking is enough. The act of asking for something and feeling desire are different animals; they are each necessary parts of the equation but one is a picture held in the mind and the other is an emotional experience. Desire itself IS one and the same with emotion, and asking is a held picture in the mind that can become action, resulting from a decision.

That said, asking can be an emotional experience also, so it's not so black and white. This process is often fraught with emotions and judgments, such as worthiness, fear, guilt, and more.

We trace pathways to a request sometimes multiple times a day. That pathway may look like this: desire->desire for something-> deciding to ask for it->asking. Taking action, including possibly asking someone for something, be it a thing or experience, is a physical experience that stems from an emotional one. In the decision-making process, will (emotions), heart, mind and spirit get involved, and that's where indecision happens, and emotion may be held instead of expressed. When that lack of flow is revealed, manifestation may not match the desire.

Desire and Faith

Another friend, Karen, presented the following counterpoint: "Perhaps in your "seeking" you have kept the experience from you because some part of you "wants" it, "yearns" for it. So the "wanting" is granted. You must *know* it's already been accomplished. In the knowing is the *is* of it. Don't ask for stuff, *know* that it's already been given."

Karen's point sounds logical enough. However, there is a subtle negating of the emotional body within the belief. Emotionality and desire reflect the Feminine Principle, which we need as deeply as we do the Masculine. In Karen's worldview, desire does not play a legitimate role in the process of manifestation; awareness is enough. Spiritually-oriented people have been afraid of the "chaos" of emotionality and in the unexamined fear of chaos have rejected desire as unnecessary and actually at cross-purposes to Spirit and the business of manifestation.

On the other hand, "knowing it *is* and then it is done" does suggest another aspect of manifestation: the need for faith that what is desired will manifest *in right timing*. If such an object of desire "is" then I can tap into my faith that I just need to open to it, and *will* open to it, in right timing. That right timing includes a possible necessity to not obtain the object of desire as soon as the self wants it, likely because further healing needs to happen in that area before fulfillment can appear. The faith that the universe will respond with exactly what you need *when you need it* is a key part of the process.

Chapter 26: Personal Empowerment

Why aren't all of us powerfully manifesting our lives in accordance with our truest hearts' desires? If desire is the key to manifestation, why do we yearn and long, in many cases for years on end, and still go unrequited? The following song may offer some clues:

Power Flower

All the ways that I'm not free
All the times I can't be me
All the lies I've told myself,
All the anger on the shelf
All the ways I haven't grown
All the chances I have blown
All the letting myself down
All the endless cycling round

Love must be allowed to heal
Love must be allowed to feel
Can you tell me how to free
These gifts that I have found in me
Love Desire Wisdom and Practicality
Love Desire Wisdom and Practicality
Love Desire Wisdom and Practicality
A power flower comes to be

Come back to me and bloom in my field
Come back to me and help me to heal

Come back to me sweet fragrances yield
A power flower

All the habits still about
All the mistrust, all the doubt
All the moments holding back
All investment in my lack
All the blaming someone else
All the acting out impulse
All the love allowed to wilt
All the listening to guilt

We must be allowed to heal
We must be allowed to feel
Can you water keep and feed
This rainbow garden's secret weed
Love Desire Wisdom and Practicality
Love Desire Wisdom and Practicality
Love Desire Wisdom and Practicality
So power flowers can grow free

Can't pry petals with my fingers
Can't force open a slow blooming rose
Yet with every feeling I move and express
Life force grounds and swells and flows

Come back to me and be as a seed
Come back to me in my hour of need
Come back to me, I need to succeed
Power flower

All the parts that I've denied
All the ruses that I've tried
All the hungers with no food
All the ghosts that I've pursued
All the judgments I have made
All intentions gone astray
All of this do I forgive
All of me I want to live

Love Desire Wisdom and Practicality
Love Desire Wisdom and Practicality
Love Desire Wisdom and Practicality
A power flower comes to be
A power flower growing free
A power flower now in me

You must have heard the phrase "I gave my power away". Many of us did give our power away. And those in the universe whose "job" it is to suck up that denied power are doing a fine job of it.

Those to whom we unconsciously give our power are the "1%", beings who for better or worse are repositories for our denied power. Each time we make a disempowered choice, one that does not come from our deepest truth, one that comes from guilt or denied fear or denied emotion of any kind, we lose a little bit of our personal power.

They use that power "against" us to "overpower" us, because we, at some early point many eons ago, judged against power as being wrong, unloving in fact. I would like to believe that overpowering in the world is simply the equivalent of a light bulb burning brighter before it burns out completely.

The judgment has since reflected to us from 'out there' as power unlovingly used. Judgments against our own inherent power –to draw desired realities toward ourselves, to keep ourselves safe, etc. – withhold our power's accessibility.

Consensus Judgments

Speaking of power, consensus judgments have incredible power. When something is accepted as "reality" by a majority of people in the world, that reality is exponentially empowered to remain manifest. As individuals, all we can do when facing classic consensus judgments in ourselves is release our particular participation in these consensus judgments (through expressing and vibrating them in sound) and feel the feelings of hopelessness and whatever else arises while attempting judgment release. Sometimes what feels like truths are really judgments in disguise, repeated and believed by so many that they take on the authority of truth. "I have no power as an individual to change things" is one example of such a judgment. Others may sound something like these:

→ "There is no changing the status quo"
→ "You have to have a lot of money to effect change"
→ "My safety is at the whim of the powers that be"
→ "I don't have any idea what to do and no knowing of how to find out".

Available power within love (power centered in the heart) fuels the power of manifestation, which is aligned with personal desire and spiritual fulfillment. True loving power does not overpower anybody or anything to meet its agenda. The power to stand firm in one's right role and place, saying yes or no with conviction is the first step on a long road back to recovering our trust for our deeper powers of manifestation and magic.

Chakras, Karmic Bonds & Cording

Once we become aware of subtle energy and how it works, we find we are often literally "bound" to others via perceivable cords of attachment extending from certain parts of our energy body to certain parts of another's. Our energy body is our auric field, consisting of several layers and including chakras, or energy centers.

Chakra is a Sanskrit word familiar to many in the alternative healing community, which translates as "wheel of light". Our energy centers or chakras are perceived through clairvoyance (or clairsentience) as subtly turning energy vortices – wheels. They exist at key points in our energy body that pertain to specific parts of the body, such as the perineum, the sacrum, the solar plexus, the center of the breastbone, the hole of the throat, the "third eye" in the middle of the forehead, and the center of our crown.

When we have cords of energy attaching to another person, there is an imbalance going on between the people involved. The energy cords illustrate the imbalance, usually indicating a flow of energy from one party to the other.

How do these imbalances occur in the first place? Some examples include unresolved issues between the people involved, denied emotions these people hold in their fields about the other person that bind them to the other, vows of debt and indenture from one to the other, judgments made about the other person.

The following was written by Seamas Manly, and is reprinted here by permission. Seamas is a Doctor of Traditional Chinese Medicine and a skilled psychic:

"When people throw anger at each other, they create strings of energy that bind them to each other. To a clairvoyant, these strings of energy look similar to a spider web. When people hurt each other, they create an energetic connection, which may bind them together over lifetimes unless and until released. If they continually repeat the same patterns with each other many times, they may have to go through many layers of healing and forgiveness in order to be free.

When people try to help other people without permission, or in a way that violates the other party's free will, they create strings of energy that bind them. This may manifest in the form of interference from other well-meaning individuals. When people use psychic gifts to pry into the lives of other people, or use energy to directly manipulate other people without their consent, they bind themselves. Some people with this pattern also have made past life vows never to be psychic again. These vows may need to be canceled in order for these people to reclaim their natural abilities.

Similarly, people with past life issues of power abuse may have made vows to never again allow themselves to be powerful. They may find themselves repeatedly in the role of victim, or of helpless bystander, until they claim the power that is their birthright. When people gossip about or internally judge other people, they bind themselves. These energetic bindings that people create may hamper their evolution in a variety of different ways, both present and future. Realizing the source of such self-imposed limitations can be both humbling and painful. People may also have lines of energy binding them to places on Earth where they participated in the polarity of aggressor/victim. Sometimes, actually visiting those places will accelerate a person's healing process through reclaiming lost essence. Most people have created thousands of these dysfunctional energetic bonds. The current state of the world is a direct reflection of this. As much rage as people have denied, there is that much mega tonnage of nuclear weapons, and that much pollution."

Releasing Karmic Cords

Getting ourselves out of these undesirable bonds is a conscious act. It may be necessary to move feelings, release judgments (review Chapter 17 for more information about how to accomplish effective judgment release), and release vows or contracts between you and the other person. It also can help to attempt detachment of these cords via a skilled energy healer who is emotions-friendly. You can also do your own ritual with a focused and conscious prayer, asking that all cords that are not yours be cut and returned to their owners and all yours be cut and returned to yourself. Doing this many times a week can help to undo unconscious cording.

To release a vow, you can start the process by formally canceling the contract you have with that person. Say out loud, "I declare the vow and contract I have with _____ null and void. I release myself and I release _____. I call all of my essence to come back to me from _____ and release any of _____'s essence I may be holding to return to her. I nullify this agreement across all time and space and realities, as well as outside time and space." If this brings up emotions for you, so much the better - let yourself express them as fully and deeply as you can, releasing as many judgments as you can find once you come up for air.

The Dark Before Dawn

The following is a poem which speaks to the issue of power and the denied power reflection from the mirror the "powers that be" are holding up to us these days from "out there." The poem calls on us to question (and eventually release) the belief that we have no responsibility for the reflection we get from our "world mirror":

Little boy blue has shit on his shoe
    And doesn't want to notice
He says, "it's you who stink
    And if you think
        We're letting you empower
Well, we'll never cower
    From a war in which we'll win
We are the masters of spin
    And this great country of ours
Despite the din from the great unheard
    Herd, will not go idly
        Into that good night.
Nope, not us...we'll fight fight fight
    Because of course, we're right
And right wins wars, and evens scores
    And more.
We say, you scurvy whore
    Battle me, and you will see
Who still steals the flower of power
    From the weak and undeserving."

Fie upon that! I'll spit in my hat
    'fore I'll go back to being
as before, when I blamed you
    as the causal bore and believed it.
Yes, that's right, I bought that bullshit
    Cuz I barely knew better.
Now it's down to me & mine
    Who are doing time
In our sheds and caves
    Riding the waves
        Of our emotions and devotions

To She who will save us.

So if you feel it,
> make a fuss, you gloomy gus,

Guilt ridden and gone from sight
> Give up going past your plight

And let's live for today
> Though it's not all play.

The row we hoe is uneven and dark
> And we are frightened
>> And our hearts
>>> Have tightened
>>>> Somewhat.

It's the dark before dawn
> So quit playing the pawn

And leave their game cuz it's
> Only the same tame shame

Join us on the edge
> Make your inner pledge

To piss or poop so to please the pot
> Before they come and throw you off

And you scream, "why me?
> The world's gone crazy, and
>> I didn't know."

Yes you did
> But you ran and hid

God help me
> Let's take responsibility
>> For being free.

True Love Power

What would true personal empowerment look like? In its most healed form, power would be an expression of true balance within us, coming from our centers, our hearts. We would deny nothing, speak our truth vulnerably, display true courage by powerfully facing our fear, expressing this fear in emotional release via sound and body movement, and taking right action in right time. We would stand up for ourselves and our loved ones without standing *against* anything or anyone, accepting what feels right to us to accept and letting the rest go. We would take responsibility for everything that happens within and to us, and we would express everything we felt in safe, responsible, and appropriate ways.

Manifesting what we need and consciously empowering others so they in turn could empower us, we would become conscious, responsible stewards of our bodies, our homes, our communities and our planet. We would begin to manifest and develop each of the powers we have lost and given up hope to ever have again, such as powers of telekinesis, telepathy, instant manifestation, bi-location, form change, and speeding up the vibration of our bodies to the speed of light at will.

To get to this ideal place of personal empowerment we must engage in healing and dealing in ways that feel right and effective for us, and not stop until we find true balance. I trust we will recognize such empowerment when we arrive.

The following was written by Nathalie St. Amant and is reprinted here with permission:

"Sometimes loss of power is very tricky and hidden within fully accepted social imprints and conditioning (consensus judgments as mentioned above). For example, one of the biggest consensus judgments I have felt enslaved by and have had to release within myself is around "what beauty is" in our society. There are cultures with different "ideas" of what that would be (containing judgments), yet the western world has [implemented] societal brainwashing with mass media, movies, musical bands, and social networking on the internet.

"For women it is a HUGE tragedy, a violent phenomenon that is barely perceived as such. A man in a film can gain a lot of popularity and be seen as attractive no matter what he looks like and we will find handsomeness in his skills or his "character". Women have a more limited field of possibility to partake in the elitism of what is called 'beauty'. I am always extremely shocked to see how deep these judgments go and how enslaved we all are by them. Women hurt themselves by accepting these perceptions as truth and men hurt themselves by dissociating from their true feelings about what truly feels beautiful to their hearts.

"On both sides we have a tragedy that is barely seen as important. Men, dissociating from love that could be seen as diversified, unique, imperfect natural beauty, are caging themselves in the addiction of reverie with these enslaving images and therefore are missing out on real, deep, mature relationships. For women, we need to learn to catch these very sticky, sneaky judgments and images, throw them out of our "house", and take responsibility for our side in this.

"In this case, empowerment would look like a more vast all- encompassing, inclusive support of different and unpredictable forms of beauty, a radical change in how separated we have all become, and a drastic shift in behaviors sprouting from competition and jealousy. Women would support each other better so communities would be held together better by that very important feminine glue.

"The more we all work on such 'impossible' consensus imprinting, the more it will become passé to engage in these old judgmental patterns, and the more we can evolve from these shockingly hidden attacks."

Our Lost Spiritual Powers

There are legends about the powers we no longer retain that are our birthright. Many psychics and spiritually oriented people remember these powers we have lost, powers that seem so fantastic and otherworldly that it is next to impossible for most of us to imagine ourselves manifesting them outside the fantasy realm.

Some of these powers include:

- Bi-location - being in two places at once.
- Teleportation - disappearing and re-appearing somewhere else
- Instant Manifestation – magically manifesting whatever is desired
- Form Change – changing our appearance at will
- Telekinesis – moving other objects without touching them.

If you are among those who believe a human being retaining and using such powers is impossible and fictional, consider the possibility of releasing the judgments you hold here. If "even bothering to do so" brings up emotions for you, it will be important to release them as described in detail in this book. Remember, all things we do not remember having seen before all through human history, things that eventually became commonplace, were ridiculed at first.

*   *   *   *   *   *   *   *

Part V

The Relational Body -

Love, Family, Friends & Others

Chapter 27: Relationships

Healing within the context of a relationship is perhaps the most challenging piece of the work we will ever do. We want a solid, committed, yummy relationship, but the road to a time-tested, work-in-progress pairing is strewn with casualties. We seem to make the same mistakes, and repeat the same patterns of behavior, reactivity, and reversal so often that it is truly amazing that we keep continuing our search for connection.

How does it come to this? After all, relationship is so incredible in the beginning. For most of us we begin in the "honeymoon phase", juicy and dreamy. Why can't it be like that forever? This part of any relationship marks the halcyon days often used as a yardstick against the fearful, guilty, angry and sad realities that can eventually replace the honeymoon phase and become the norm with our loved one. Distancing or fighting creeps in, overlaying the effortless connectedness we had so enjoyed before.

We are not necessarily projecting perfection in the beginning, or overlooking all the bad stuff, although that may sometimes be the case. It is just that in the very beginning, we have not yet found the gap

The Gap

As we ascend to the heights of the honeymoon stage, we also cut deeper, in exact measure. We grow in all ways within a relationship, separately and together; the energy of the "relationship entity" or the combined field of the two people involved quite literally gets bigger. This energy pushes on all the unhealed and unexamined places within ourselves and our partner, and "the gap" is the container for all that we had previously pushed away and anything we resist looking at too closely.

The gap is another word for splits or holes in our energy field, and into those subconscious gaps go everything we have not dealt with or consciously accepted. The gap is always lurking within us, until we are completely healed, and it cannot be avoided when interpersonal connections get deeper and begin to touch our places of wounding. The gap is within us as individuals and between us as couples.

The gap is primarily a time gap. The time between receiving a trigger and expressing natural emotional response to that trigger can be minutes, hours, years or lifetimes-long. The longer the time gap, the longer and more powerfully my denial is able to affect me and those around me in potentially destructive ways.

The following commentary further explaining the gap was written by Kendra Thomas and is reprinted here by permission:

"The gap is not logical because the gap is the disconnected part of Self, disconnected from conscious awareness and understanding of the now. It holds a faulty core belief that was actually true in the moment for that reality when this part of you split off from the rest, but that faulty core belief is held frozen and cannot evolve.

That part of you appears illogical but it actually is very logical if you go ask it what it thinks and why, and allow it to tell you its story. Then you can see why that part of you would think that way. Then of course feeling and expressing the feelings is what brings in Spirit, which is understanding, and gets that part of you caught up with events and understandings of the here and now.

The gap is in your own subconscious mind where the unexpressed feelings from the past are disconnected from the current understandings of the now."

Different people handle hitting the gap in different ways. Some of us act out, engaging in addictive behaviours of escape. Some of us blame our partner to avoid taking responsibility for our part. At our best, we can learn to recognize and apply the understanding that our partner is our mirror, showing us something we cannot yet see or accept about ourselves. Getting this, we seek in our healing intent amidst the emotional turmoil to find our role or responsibility in the situation.

When in a gap, dropping out of words as soon as possible and into wordless emotional release minimizes damage to the hearts involved. The gap's arrival is signaled by a surface trigger. In response to this trigger, one person or both people in the relationship surfaces old, sometimes ancient emotional pain. When the gap is present, this pain is not recognized as emanating from within the self. Instead it looks like the mirror, or "other" is the cause and source of this pain. We are sure they have done something to us, and need to apologize or change.

It can take a big effort to be consciously aware enough to remind ourselves: "it's about me, I know it's really about me", when the initial translation of the rising feeling is actually most often, "Dammit I KNOW IT'S ABOUT THEM!!!"

If I am able to cry my hurt or express my anger or fear appropriately, space can be cleared within the receptive centers of the emotional body, and spirit can enter that space with the light of understanding. I then can receive realizations about my own involvement. "Ohhhhh....THAT'S what it's really about...THIS is where I come in... this is what s/he is reminding me of...yeahhhhhh". The more I express the triggered feelings in sound or in tears and heal my hurt places, the more I do not have these triggers so "in my face" that I am flailing and blindly striking back and blaming. In fact, once true depth of understanding is reached, these kinds of overwhelming triggers are no longer drawn by the emotional body, which only draws an exact energetic match to the size of the emotional energy that is being held in a state of denial regarding the issue at hand.

It helps to deeply examine the belief many of us carry that says "If I am right, I win and I feel good/If I am wrong, I will die". The battle for right and wrong is a red herring. I can slice and dice in a point of view battle with anyone. But winning this kind of war is a lonely victory. My mate is either bruised or bleeding afterwards. So am I if I look closely enough, though my heart is probably too closed to care, until I can open again and see the cost of my "win".

A Key: Seeking My Responsibility

When I feel victimized, I can ask myself, what subconscious or split-off part of me is drawing this reflection to me? Our split-off, unowned (aka "gapped") energies draw situations to ourselves that can be triggers for balancing those energies. One of the most difficult aspects of a given gap between lovers is recognizing the interlocking and meshing patterns that are enacted between the two. They are often complex and disguised, or completely hidden, especially when strong feelings are being stirred into life.

When things reach the point in a relationship where I cannot tell what is going on, who started what or who is responsible, I have found that the easiest way out of the morass is to seek my own responsibility. I have also found that it is a losing proposition to instead speculate aloud upon my partner's responsibility or blame them for what I am sure they are "doing wrong".

I prefer to feel, and express, whatever it is I feel, in a safe and responsible way, and then look at what my role is – because most often the understanding is not available until after the emotions stirred are resolved, particularly if I start with any kind of blaming, angry feelings toward my partner. If I try to figure it out either in my own brain first or in charged dialogue with my partner during the emotional activation phase of the gap, I do not get very far. Once I express and the fog clears, I can more easily see my responsibility.

Letting Go

Sometimes I notice that even after emotionally expressing, receiving understandings and feeling better, my partner is still acting out. Rather than try to change, stop, pressure or control my partner, if I can now clearly see her behavior for what it is, I can move back from her as a way to set a self-loving boundary until cooler heads prevail. When the charge has receded enough I can "come back to the table", so to speak, and communicate my side of responsibility for the trigger at hand. I can offer my own commitment for change on my end.

Doing so can often lead by example, for I have become willingly vulnerable by sharing what I perceive my responsibility to be, and perhaps she too will feel organically encouraged by my actions to follow suit. If she does not, it is not healing and dealing for me to coerce or cajole her. My power in the situation is to share my side and either move back from any ongoing behavior that does not work for me, or negotiate for the win-win if it feels like right time to try for that. Possibly I have become clearer about any boundaries I might have or need to state than when I was carrying a lot of emotionally reactive charge.

Why do we keep going toward finding functional relationship? Perhaps it is the potential of self-awareness and the desire to apply it, live it, and return to a deeper phase of the honeymoon stage, to match the original dreams and visions of a match made in the heaven of our hearts.

Chapter 28: Interactive Process

When triggered by another in your space, move away from them when possible, unless the two of you have a longstanding agreement or unwritten "contract" to do this kind of interpersonal work together. Are you each willing to feel the "cascade" of back'n'forth triggering along with the leaking blame that inevitably spews? Doing the emotional work necessary to eventually get to the place where you can take responsibility for your involvement in each and every controversy is crucial.

"I Need To Spew"

I have made a big deal of saying that expressing emotions such as anger in pure sound (i.e. wordless sound) is the best and deepest way to go to fully release it. To get to this point, beginning this process in words is sometimes necessary. What my partner and I say about the sort of unwritten/unspoken "contract" to do this work together, is "I need to spew". A spew, for us, is intended to get us all the way over to wordless flashpoint/ignition.

Sometimes the hateful, angry, blaming, controlling words are needed as bridges to get us all the way to the primal rage that has no words. Saying "I need to spew" is a sort of magic short-circuit of the blaming and avoidance that acting out unconsciously produces. Spewing is done not as a way to get away with pounding someone else and making it "their fault", but rather as a way for each of us to find our flashpoint of primal expression. Spewing as consciously as possible under the circumstances enables us to notice that, "I need to get these words out of me, because in this scenario, they are acting as a cork on my deeper feelings." In this way, spewing is used as a tool toward achieving personal responsibility.

I sometimes spew in private, away from the trigger, especially if the other person is not willing to have me spew in their presence, or if my emotional body does not feel safe enough in the moment with this person. Most often it works best in the presence of the trigger, but only if that person is an emotional "mover" with an understanding of what I am doing. This is a very specialized scenario. It can be helpful to note often during a "spewing session" that I am doing just that, spewing in order to get the harsh or angry words out of me, so other people don't get the notion that I am really trying to blame them or make them wrong.

Virtual Process

Interactive process via email can be a real minefield. There are, of course, many layers to utilizing interpersonal process via email. These are a few of the basic tenets that I have seen to work (and not work) in over twenty years of doing online process in groups and 1-1. "E-rage" can be an issue in cyber communications, and most often the ways e-rage has been being used is not healing and dealing, but another form of acting out.

When feeling triggered by what someone says in an email, I take a moment and drop my hands from the keyboard, close my eyes, and feel into my solar plexus. Do I feel a swirling of feelings that might be able to emerge in sound if I walked away from the computer? Yes? I then let it loose right there, or go off somewhere else, and come back to the computer some other time, when I have integrated enough, and let the person know (if they are someone I feel safe sharing this with). To me, these are the "safe triggers" that do not have to be stirred by a major event outside me.

Did I get some understandings from that movement, something I can share with the person who triggered me? Did I find a deeper layer that transcended the surface trigger, some more ancient story? Did I find some personal responsibility that I feel motivated to share? Something that is not about the triggering person, but about me? I have found that this latter piece in particular disarms a war in progress, be it a small or large war. Ways that I have responsibility for the current skirmish are crucial to discover so that effective healing and dealing can be enacted.

There is always a kernel of truth in a printed rage spew, but it is nearly impossible to gracefully receive with the undercurrents that ride along. These are undercurrents inherent in the backlog of old anger coming up in the triggered person that has not moved yet, which in many cases has nothing to do with the other person but everything to do with the enraged person's history and what is being currently triggered in them

Acceptance, A Key to Safe Expression

Acceptance, as opposed to lack of acceptance, makes all the difference in how expressed emotion feels to all concerned. To truly accept emotion, one must cultivate a general understanding that the emotion s/he is feeling is *theirs*, not the "fault" of somebody else. Pure expression does not act out in fights, words, threats or destruction. Pure emotional expression of hurt, rage, terror, or grief, is in wordless sound and tears, exerting minimal control on what sounds are released and maximal control on acting out behaviours. Primal emotional expression, along with physical touch, when appropriate, is always the shortest distance between two hearts.

Chapter 29: Reflections and Personal Responsibility

"As without, so within". Imagine a whole universe inside us. What does that really mean, and how can that awareness help us heal? Are we not just organic tissue and fluids inside?

Assuming that there are more realms of existence than the physical, everything we know to exist outside ourselves exists at some level of our inner being. Everything we participate with outside us, we participate with inside, and it follows that everything that happens to us experientially is going on inside us already, perhaps at the subconscious levels of existence.

No Accidents: Our ElectroMagnetic Nature

If there is a reason for everything that happens to me, and if I create my own reality, then there are no such things as accidents, coincidences, random occurrences and "luck". The magnetic power in my emotional body draws to me the precise experiences I need in order to learn and evolve, and draws the experiences I need to release the latent personal power trapped in my subconscious.

Do you believe everything happens for a reason, or that nothing happens to us by chance? Biological beings are electromagnetic in nature. We have an electric side and a magnetic side. Our electric side is our yang selves, our doing, acting selves, the masculine polarity/left brain/right sides of who we each are regardless of gender. And our yin, receiving, accepting sides are our magnetic sides, the left side/right brain, the feminine. Yin energy has just as much power as yang, but it is an indrawing power. Our feminine sides, our magnetic selves, draw necessary learning and healing experiences. Our electromagnetism explains why we do not live in a random universe.

We draw, or magnetize, exactly what we need to experience in order to grow. And this is why, even if I can't see it, even if something "justifiably" enrages me, I know I have some responsibility for drawing it to my reality. This is how I "create" my own reality, regardless of whether I like or am conscious of what I have created. I only "choose" my reality consciously insofar as my magnetic/emotional essence is conscious. Often these parts are subconscious due to being chronically denied, but still consist of magnetic emotional essence drawing realities to me. Here, consciousness is "out of the loop" and that hidden part of the brain known as the subconscious is responsible for drawing an experience I didn't consciously see coming.

Despite our lack of awareness that our subconsciousness draws experiences to us, we can still accept that this subconscious magnetic essence in us is loving. This hidden part of ourselves draws these experiences to us in exact proportion to the level of emotional backlog we have. We draw the strength or intensity of experience that we require in order to bring ourselves to balance by finally, this time, not ignoring and instead accepting how we really feel about what is happening to us. This is so we can heal (i.e. bring to balance) what we have previously ignored or glossed over. Once we have sufficient experiences in a given issue and process all the resultant feelings in response, layer by layer, we eventually become able, or response-able, to understand and own the root cause so deeply we no longer have to experience anything so relatively harsh again in order to learn about ourselves in a particular area.

Many of us are so electric in so much of our consciousness that when we have not actively executed an action that would create an outcome, we tell ourselves we could not have had responsibility. Culturally we are still in the process of learning that magnetic essence draws experiences "out of thin air". This is how pain is self-created (though never consciously desirable).

Most people, however, do not accept this as a truth. We feel justified in blaming others because when "they do it to me" it is all "their fault" and none of ours. When in blame, we are righteous victims only. This is a distortion our world has been running on since the beginning. The truth buried in unexpressed emotions "underneath" the blame can give us significant clues as to where our responsibility lies. But, in most cases, we cannot access it unless those emotions are vibrated. In order to come to balance in any given conflict, we must first intend to discover what our responsibility is.

Human Magnets

Pleasant experiences reflect the accepted, vibrating, conscious parts of self; unpleasant ones reflect the unaccepted, non-vibrating, unconscious parts. When we draw pleasant experiences, we feel joy, enthusiasm, passion, etc. and hopefully we express those -- they are just as important to accept and express as the hard feelings. With unpleasant ones we are likewise called upon to express our true response, when we feel sadness, grief, irritation, anger, rage, hurt, fear or terror. When we do not express our natural emotional response, we will draw to ourselves a more intense experience than last time. The magnetic essence, just a little more intensely denied and impacted than it was, now needs a stronger experience in order to overcome resistance and trigger itself into life. Living things have varying degrees of vibration, and dead things have little to no vibration. The dead parts of ourselves, judged so long ago to be unacceptable and wrong, can come back to life, but until we un-deny (accept) them, they sit still in the dark, awaiting acceptance for the treasure they have to offer.

Because of chronic and imprinted patterns of denial, we have been cut off from the awareness of the power we have, consciously or subconsciously, to magnetize EVERYTHING that happens to us. A car crash I experienced in 1985 is certainly nothing I would have consciously chosen to manifest. At that time my subconscious denial was so massive and so in control of what I was manifesting that it needed to draw a huge and dramatic experience such as a head-on collision with a drunk driver. I can see in hindsight that I needed an experience of this order of magnitude to get me off the dime toward a choice to intentionally heal what was buried in my subconscious. I drew this experience without knowing what I was doing, or why.

The more unconscious my denial is, the more the experience it draws to trigger itself seems random and the more victimized I feel. The part of me drawing an experience that harsh is literally unconscious. It took a lot of process and deep personal inquiry for me to connect to my magnetic responsibility, not only for this car crash but for everything that happens to me. In this example, all I felt was victimized until I realized this magnetic connection I have to the events which seem to "randomly" happen to me.

At first we cannot understand or explain why something happens to us because the core reasons are buried in the subconscious. Within the subconscious layers of our brain live old, denied emotions, separated from awareness. We can only recover this awareness piece by piece by "vibrating" or allowing the trapped emotions to rise and show our conscious selves what they have been holding. My experiences show me where I am denying, insofar as I do not understand what they are showing me -- they are "reflecting" to me, holding up a mirror, of what I am not currently seeing (as well as whatever portion of it I already do understand). Deciphering the reflections is an art form and becomes easier the more I practice and the more experience I gain.

The entire reason for drawing the new experience is to trigger the held emotion and gain resulting awareness and understanding about why I had a similar, original experience way back in the beginning, in my very first incarnation as a manifested being. Drawing the new experience triggers the held emotion that connects us with similar previous experiences in this life and then helps us unfold deeper levels of memories in past lives all the way back to when the trauma originated (sometimes all the way back to our very first incarnation) Once I gain the fullest, deepest understanding I can get on a particular issue, I no longer have to repeat the same kind of unpleasant experience and can finally move on to more pleasant evolutionary experiences. I will only know for sure that "I'm done" with a given issue when similar types of experiences cease, or cease to trigger me. They often start detaching from us and can become things that happen to others around us. We can recognize the pattern now with the greater perspective that distance offers, until it is completely cleared.

Let's say somebody hits me after shouting at me and threatening me. I have somehow brought this on myself, because, well, "I create everything in my own reality". Sounds good, but it feels bad. Why? Because there is more to the picture than that.

Yes, I have a dynamic inside me that is indeed drawing this "reflection" of my inner turmoil. But it takes at least two to create an interpersonal incident. My abuser is the active party in the incident, and s/he has responsibility for the action s/he has taken. But I too have responsibility for drawing an *exact, energetic match* to the unreleased rage and terror trapped within my subconscious, in a *state of denial*.

Because this energy is denied, it is not conscious. Because it is not conscious, it is not controllable. Emotional energy is magnetic and draws to itself the exact experience necessary to bring release. If someone is hitting me, I have an equivalent energetic charge inside me that matches the outer reflection in precise proportion. I need these reflections to learn about what I am holding, and why I am holding it, so I can release it instead of continuing to deny it inside me.

The most effective way I have found to draw more pleasant experiences is to safely release emotions, either with myself or with a trusted healing partner. I do this by expressing the emotions in sound, without hurting myself or anyone else. I use pillows to beat, scream or cry into. I allow fear to express in keening wails or simply let my jaw chatter.

We can ameliorate the "negative intensity" of our experiences if we are proactive about our emotional state and what we have denied since we were little children. Emotional expression is tied into personal power, and if we deny our power, it will "reflect" outside ourselves as power in a state of denial working against us. Taking responsibility in this context means feeling deeply into what our experiences say about what we have been holding onto and ignoring for a very long time, and doing something about it. That might simply be feeling what we feel. When we can be mindful of this, then we can watch our reflections shift to more of what we like and less of what we do not.

The Parts We Left Behind

This is a song to all of my brothers out there
And as sometimes I will, I come now to say to beware
Not to every Body, but if you're some Body
Then maybe you've ears that can hear

Starts with intention to go back in misty old time
Parts of us there
Were committing unspeakable crimes
Don't you know we're still hurting
From all of that skirting
Responsibility we left behind

If we own our perpetrator, our inner woman hater,
Then maybe true healing we'll find
We've got to own our child abuser,
And the parts that casually use her
Then maybe we'll stop being blind
From denials which kill us in kind
In the parts of us we left behind

This is a song to all of my sisters out there
And as sometimes I have,
I come now to say to take care
With all of the crying, and all of the dying
It's all been the same, but now things can change

For they've been killing our will to live,
They've been killing our need to give
They've been killing our creativity,
They've been killing our space for nativity

They've refused us the right to say 'no',
They want us dead but they don't let it show
 "They" are us in a brilliant disguise,
In the mirrors we don't recognize

Rage rage to bring the coming of the light
Rage rage to bring the ending of the night
Safe safe release can make it right
Shake shake tremble and quake
Scream and shout, a hellish noise make

This is a song to compassionate hearts just like me
When we say it ain't us,
Well, we might as well cut down the trees
Can't be scared to show fear,
That the end might be near
And what we don't know can hurt us, it's clear

If we own our perpetrator, our inner woman hater,
Then maybe true healing we'll find
We've got to own our child abuser,
And the parts that casually use her
Then maybe we'll stop being blind
From denials which kill us in kind
In the parts of us we left behind

Chapter 30: Competition - A Dog Eat God World

"The guy's a fierce competitor...hates losing...great to watch him play." Sound like the description of any athletes you have read about or known? The competitive drive, while all well and good in the structured, rules-centric arena of sports events, can be destructive between friends, family members, co-workers and lovers. "Competition has its place, but NIMBY (not in my back yard)."

The drive to come out on top, to be right, to sell the most widgets, or to have the best spot is one we all struggle with sometimes. Some of us deny that we have such a drive, always giving over to somebody else who wants what we want. Others, talented and experienced at competing and quicker than most, take everything they can every chance they get, trumpeting "I got here first, to the winner go the spoils".

We want to be right so we can feel good about ourselves; we tell ourselves we like to debate or are good at winning arguments. We also want to be right so we can avoid feeling wrong, which deep inside can equate to feeling bad about ourselves, unworthy, and even endangered. "If I am wrong, what will happen to me?"

Some of the most beautiful epiphanies in life are when we can admit to one we were competing with that we made a mistake or were out of line, without making ourselves wrong for having done so. Humble moments following the heat of battle (either subtle or overt) are paradoxically moments of great strength and love.

Judgments Driving Competition

Looking under the hood, we see several root beliefs and imprints causing us to repeatedly and habitually dip into the chaotic waters of competition. The scarcity judgment many hold is a big issue. "There isn't enough, so I better go get mine now before s/he does". People with a sense of entitlement are oft-admired. Yet this sense can come by these people having competed ruthlessly and won, then forgotten having done so. Worse, these folks sometimes may engage in justifying past competitive behavior by blaming, belittling or finding fault with the vanquished in some way. These may be folks who as children or young adults were never taught limits or boundaries around overriding others to get what they want. Or, they had things given to them without being taught the need to appreciate what abundance is and from whence it comes.

Nearly every strong feeling we experience gets stirred by hidden or overt competition, whether we like competing or not. In order to balance the reality of living in a competitive world we have to come to terms with these feelings and express them fully. The cost of denying how we really feel about competing, why we compete or do not compete, and what drives all of it is that we will continue to draw triggering competition scenarios until we end the denial of our feelings.

Ultimately, we need to reveal these feelings to ourselves, God, Earth Mother or Great Spirit, whomever we call Deity. We need to show how we really feel underneath the desperate need to be right all the time, or about lack of love, money or resources. We need to show

how we really feel about "living in a dog eat dog world". Are we enraged at The Divine or The Universe for not bringing enough? Getting real, we can gain understanding about how we can come to balance with these heavy issues.

Competition, blame and fighting come from the part of the brain called "reptilian". The reptilian brain's function is to operate automatically as a temporary shield when the body is being traumatized or attacked in moments when Body cannot yet handle the situation in a safe way. This shielding is accomplished without emotional heart presence.

The problem is that this part of the brain should function in balance with the limbic part of the brain that supplies the emotional heart. Our emotional heart ideally feels, heals and deals with any situation. However, the emotional part of the brain and body is underdeveloped and has been oppressed in western culture. This is the part of the brain that allows us to drop from the fight or flight and the I AM RIGHT reptilian brain mechanism into a self-responsible, vulnerable, loving, healing, inner child place. In the world as we know it, the reptilian brain rules our lives in large part. It has become urgent that we heal and deal in a way that can bring this part of our brains back into balance, which in the macrocosm will end war.

Chapter 31: Strong Emotions Around Children

Belief systems around emotional healing get passed down through the generations, and one major belief is that strong emotions need to be hidden from children so as to not damage them. This belief has, in part, arisen from how emotions traditionally have been expressed: wild, blaming fights between parents, the destruction of property, threatening and controlling rage in the form of words delivered directly in the faces of children, etc.

The emotions in these cases are "breaking loose"; that is, overcoming the inner restraints on their expression with the strength of their pent-up charge. In this, there is a subconscious intent to get rid of the pain instead of owning and really feeling it. Since in countless cases there is no acceptance for loud emotion taking any form at all, with the unspoken inner mandate to hold back if at all possible, these emotions are literally expressing unacceptably. The people involved are acting out the emotions instead of directly expressing their charge with self-acceptance.

Children Learn 24/7

Children take in many subtle messages from their parents' behavior, always learning even when we do not know they are. They also don't have the filters we have taken on, and can detect emotional subtleties we adults are not privy to. When we hold back a strong emotion because we judge that to be safer than expressing it in their presence, we are teaching denial of emotional expression when emotions rise, and children absorb that teaching very specifically, albeit non-mentally, from all the cues and clues from their parents.

Mechanics of Expressing Around Kids

Next time you are angry, even if your child is the trigger, consider turning away from the child and expressing the sound in grunts or wordless yells (or better still, take a time out for yourself and head for some private space). S/he will likely be afraid or triggered also; it's alright. Let your child(ren) have these feelings in response to you, and model healthy expression of your emotions instead of modeling denial or unhealthy expression. In the right moment, in and around your expression, release judgments out loud, in words, as to how much this is going to damage your child and make everything worse, as well as any other judgments you can release about your emotional expression. Children "get" our intent, and if at first they reflect your non-acceptance of your own emotional expression (children being inherently reflective of parental denials and judgments) they will shift if you can be consistent and come to accept your own appropriate existence as an emotionally flowing human.

Sometimes emotional expression needs to start in words. One key is to turn your body away from the child and stay in words only as long as necessary to get to the "primal" level of pure sound underneath. Go to another room if preferable, and close the door. If they want to come in, let *them* determine the distance from you and your expression that feels right to them. Do not deny yourself emotionally in favor of your child if at all possible.

Deep judgments many parents hold in this area requiring formal release include:

→ "I will hurt my child with my emotional outburst. "

→ "Emotional expression is damaging, especially to children"

→ "My parents could not hold it in, and I got hurt as a result, so it's safer for my kids if I hold it in."

→ "I just do not have time or space to express myself as fully or intensively as I really feel – I have to remain functional and "there" for them at all times."

→ "My loud sound will scare them too badly and that's bad, I cannot allow my child to be scared of my sound or me"

Allowing Children To Feel Afraid

Finding terror of another's rage is a good and necessary trigger too. Children need to be allowed to have their fear response of their parents' anger without it shutting down the parent. Let children feel their terror when their parent is moving rage appropriately. Cultivate a trust that all feelings are appropriate and necessary or they would not be happening, including your children's, and let the chips fall where they may. It may feel difficult and frightening to allow everyone's feelings to be and express because this kind of natural expression is not what you or they are used to. Remind yourself at these times that continuing to teach denial by example is worse.

It's important to process whatever feelings of fear your child experiences with the child following any incident. Help them to understand that your feelings are about you and not about them, and that you'd never intentionally hurt your child.

   We parents have been invested and habituated in protecting our kids from feeling their triggers fully. We get scared by their expressions of terror because their expressions are so vital, so unencumbered. Those of us scared by these reflections are terrified of our own inner child's unprocessed fear. Fear of one's own fear is the biggest block I have seen to emotions-friendly people really getting down into the sub-levels of emotional backlog. Faith that we will make it out alive if we dare explore our terror backlog, and release of judgments around recovery from the fear expression are two keys here.

   Anger and terror can subtly act out in the form of unnecessarily controlling our children. Instead of enforcing compliance with a heavy commanding energy, we as parents are called upon sometimes to express the feelings our children trigger in us. The more emotional responsibility we can model for our children, the greater responsibility and freedom they will manifest and be able to model for the world they inherit.

Chapter 32: Children Expressing Emotions

There is very little in the world that brings a parent's triggers to the surface as quickly as the tears or loud, angry expressions of their child. Consider that much of what is seen to be your child's emotional expression may not be theirs at all. It may be yours, the parent's, refracted through the "lens" of your child's emotional body.

When I was young my father was convinced that I was doing or saying certain things or expressing in certain ways deliberately, just to upset him. I never was, but whatever it was at those moments that I was expressing or enacting never failed to trigger him with pinpoint accuracy, as if I *was* doing it intentionally. None of this was conscious for me; I was always shocked when he reacted that way. I was "just being a kid"; in other words, acting instinctively and impulsively most of the time. A certain dynamic was apparent; I was either acting out or expressing the very feelings he wanted to avoid.

Emotional Sponges

Children are little emotional sponges, exponentially more so than the most sensitive adult empath. Because of genetic and karmic linkups with the parents, they absorb, act out and reflect the very feelings we as parents have literally shoved out of ourselves, whether consciously or not, or recently or not. Imagine these denied feelings as splinters energetically entering the auric field of a psychically open child. Like physical splinters, these feelings must work their way out again, so that their rightful owners can experience and take responsibility for them in one way or another. Unfortunately, it does not always work that way, as children are often controlled out of these natural expulsions and forced to continue to try to hold these feelings.

Our Feelings, Their Feelings

In addition to this phenomenon, in many if not all cases, our children literally come into the world holding our denials already, transmitted in the sexual exchange that led to conception. Sexual exchange involves a sharing of our essence with our partners, which includes the entire gamut from love to denials. Parents have great responsibility to recover their denied parts and emotions from their children, in right timing and in an organic manner via the natural unfolding of their own healing process.

When emotions rightfully belong to the child, it is somewhat simpler. It still behooves the parents to teach appropriate expression of feelings, such as helping children remember the difference between acting out and expressing safely in sound and body movements without hurting themselves or anything/anybody else (I say "remember" because children as babies and toddlers were naturally appropriate expressers before societal and subtle internal and external pressures caused their pure expression to warp into act-out behavior). In these cases, if there are no generalized parental rules against expression, then compassion, guidance and allowance can enter and the child can offload safely and effectively. A parent can easily tell the difference as to whose emotions the child is expressing/acting out by whether s/he is triggered by their child's display of them. Of course, it is possible that in some cases, the child may be expressing their own emotion that reflects a like emotion in the parent.

Several tips for parents who are triggered by their child's actions and expressions were outlined in the previous chapter. The more completely a parent can take responsibility for the feelings that come up for them in response to their child's feelings, especially if the parent can express these feelings him or herself shortly following the trigger, the more dramatically the child's behavior can shift. I watched this happen often with my own son – when he triggered me and I was able to express my response fully in my own emotional body, he would either no longer trigger me that way with similar future behavior or would simply cease that behaviour. Pretty magical, yet simple and effective (over time) when the dynamic is accepted and applied.

The younger your child is when you decide to start being more real with your emotional expression around them, the easier it is for her to adapt to the "new normal" of emotions being expressed in sound by adults around them. Children over the age of seven may have a more challenging time adjusting to changes in how their caregivers deal with emotions. Communicating in age-appropriate ways to help your children adjust to a more emotionally expressive you will be very important for older kids – they will need your help to understand why you are suddenly allowing this expression a lot more.

Children Expressing In Public

My friend Karen responded after hearing some of this rationale for allowing children to express without heavy controls on the expression. She specifically addressed the issue of children expressing in public venues: "Yes, a baby's a ball of sound but remember the "joy" that bundle brings to a plane full of people when she is unhappy on board."

Indeed, it pushes on our own similar or identical held feelings we may have been holding since we were back at that baby's age, about when we were shushed, joggled and in a myriad of overt and subtle ways made to stop "fussing" by our parents, especially in public situations. Our raw feelings at that age were not acceptable to the outside world -- in the form of our closest contacts, no less! -- and as we grew older, we internalized that pressure to repress any emotions that tried to rise. (Still, even babies are not mere victims of their parents, in this context. If we take it as a given that this really is not our first and only life, then the beings newly reincarnated have responsibility for unresolved feelings and judgments held over from many past lives. This reality, although an extreme concept for some to embrace, allows us to recognize our personal responsibility for that which happens to us from outside ourselves, at any age. The paradox is that we are not capable at that age of taking responsibility for our feelings or reflections and shouldn't be expected to). We often label these raw feelings childish, as if feeling as acutely as a child does and being that sensitive is something reprehensible and something to outgrow, as if the relative emotional numbness of an adult is a preferable state of being.

As adults, when feelings arise or are triggered deeply enough to overcome the walls of restraint and burst loose anyway, we scramble to regain control quickly. When we begin to heal our emotional past and reach a critical mass of inner self-acceptance, these feelings and responses to outer stimuli, such as crying babies on airplanes gradually become more easily seen and accepted for what they are: an opportunity to take responsibility for our response and discover what our reaction means about us, rather than "blaming the reflection".

If a child or baby is sounding off in expression and it bothers me, and the sound might be hurting my ears, I hopefully have integrated the habit of having good earplugs nearby for such spontaneous occasions. Another possible reason it might bother me is because I have those very emotions denied and locked away somewhere, only (in this example) I do not like to be reminded of them by their external reflection in the form of a baby crying. This response occurs at a very visceral and non-mental level.

This feeling usually translates as 'ooo yuck I hate that sound, shut that kid up'. The internal recoil at being reminded is because when we were that age, we were shut down for similar behavior, and we have not processed the feelings around being shutdown yet. Nor have we processed the actual, original feelings themselves that caused our own infant selves to sound off in the first place, just like the baby on the airplane!

In Part 2: The Emotional Body, I spoke about being afraid of my own anger. When I had not yet gotten deeply into my denied rage backlog, having recently begun my exploration of my old emotions, I began to notice more closely when other people were angry -- *I just could not stand to be around them*, or even experience them at all in their irritation. Just being around them when they were irritated, or on the edge of "losing it" made me feel awful and squirmy inside.

At that time, I was deeply terrified of my anger backlog, and I could not bear to see it reflected from anywhere nearby. I was still so repressive and judgmental of my own denied anger boiling below that I had not dealt with. This anger backlog had been inexorably rising up like a Leviathan from the deep, now that I had unlocked the door in my neophyte healing process -- swung it open....CREEEEEEEAAAAAAKKKKK...imagine the terror of entering a haunted house all by yourself, and the picture is complete.

The magic of emotional expression allows the fear, grief and old rage, once expressed and integrated, to transform into trust for self, trust for triggers, and trust for the process, and the haunted house of the unexplored past transposes into a dimly lit series of rooms that can be illuminated at will.

Back to bundle screaming holy hell on the plane - I am all for a babe in arms being taken out of a movie theatre or a play or some kind of performance where the sound is interfering with others' enjoyment of the entertainment, until that baby is complete with its expression, so that the actual transmission of creativity from player to audience can be achieved. On a plane, a baby cannot be removed from the scene, and certainly feelings are legitimate in the person who feels their reading, movie or sleep is interrupted by the sound. The more we can express our own feelings of babyhood victimization when triggered or remembered, the less we will be negatively affected by such a scenario played out by a baby in our space.

In general, if we're all just sitting there "enjoying the peace and quiet", as in the cabin on an airplane - well, that peace and quiet has come at a price - the price of emotions' imprisonment via denial.

True Versus Artificial Peace

The price of any peace and quiet around us in the world as it is today is in part the price of enforced denial. In its current gestalt, the price of any peace and quiet around us is the price of other people's feelings being made to shut up (by ourselves, by others, by threat of recrimination) to afford what I would label, in many cases, *artificial* peace and quiet. The peace and quiet is artificial because if expression is being repressed to achieve it, it is not real peace. There is internal war present, just disguised and forcibly pushed outside conscious awareness, *even if we have forgotten that we have done so.*

At this stage in the overall healing of people on Earth, within this urgent need to be in touch with everything inside us that has not been emotionally processed, peace and quiet becomes the aberration. Healing and dealing emotionally, with plentiful and regular expressions of emotional sounds then becomes the norm, until the collective backlog has been dealt with and we as a race find the wherewithal to once and for all transform our global, cultural and individual patterns and imprints.

I believe we will not have *real*, abundant, and balanced peace until all internal war and internal/external overpowering has left this planet. Any peace in the interim is borrowed or illusory, and if it ends abruptly during an airplane flight, then so be it, that is a reflection of where we are at. I for one on such an airplane accept the break in silence, because noise needs to be given some space to be, to exist (emotionally primal, expressive noise, not the noise of emotions acting out) and if it is not appropriate adult expression, then a baby's wherewithal to spontaneously express will fill that role of embodying the inner signpost to what is underneath the borrowed peace. I do suggest carrying good earplugs anywhere one may go in public so as to prevent or minimize physical/auditory pain from others' expressions.

I am not meaning to convey that I "enjoy" the sound of a baby screaming on an airplane, but the expression does not push on me, perhaps because I give a lot of free space and allowance to my own emotionally-based sound, and appreciate others being given/allowing themselves the opportunity as well, when it arises. At another level you could say I *do* enjoy it, in terms of the satisfaction of noticing and knowing, "ahhhh, yet another person with emotion that needs expression is getting allowed to have it and express it, yeah, right on". I internally applaud any pure expression of the feminine/emotional vibration, even of the gnarly, painful variety, because this world contains much gnarly pain, and we need to get very real with that in order for things to really change.

Worse Before It's Better

Regarding allowing and encouraging emotionality in our children -- it may *look* for a while that it is getting worse, instead of better, as our children begin to be given some bounded green light energy to express. Any child may blow through a big piece of their backlog fairly quickly and show obvious shifts after a fairly short while. They may learn to become appropriate soon, or not so soon. There is no predicting the course of things; each child is a unique individual and the results they will get cannot be boxed into a set of definitively predictable outcomes. There is no well-mapped out course of what an individual's healing path is going to look like.

When a child begins to be encouraged to safely express, they can become the outlet for the rest of the children and adults in the house, if none are already joining her there. It might look like they are just endlessly angry and seem to have more and more and more anger as they become the literal outlet or lightning rod, so to speak, for the old, denied rages, terrors, and grief of all who are not joining the one expressing in appropriate private expression of their own. That would not be wrong, though it would not necessarily happen that way either.

Parents releasing judgments about their child's arc of expressive evolution and what it means in any individual situation that your child is expressing in a certain way is a very helpful, demonstrable tool in aiding your children to move through their backlog as quickly and efficaciously as possible. For a review on judgment release, please turn to Chapter 17: *Judgment Release*.

The Family Lightning Rod

Families are units, organisms; within a household, everyone in a family swims in the same psychic soup, in addition to the fact that they are all so similar genetically. To a degree, this dynamic shifts for family members who move away, who are no longer swimming in the same soup. This soup may be said to be a household gestalt, a particular energy that informs everyone who lives there.

If the parents are holding back a ton, the kids will express their parents' stuff in addition to their own. Parents' held back emotional energy may well leak through the children. Children do not deny as well yet as the parents, so this absorbed emotional energy shows up more in act outs, and even just crying a lot, for some kids. Children in nuclear families have their own sets of tendencies that I want to be careful to set aside as different from adults' tendencies, especially when emotional expression is concerned.

Being a lightning rod for the family's backlog is the price a child pays for exercising her Divine right (and I do not use that expression lightly) of being allowed to be a kid fully expressing her own rage safely with parental encouragement and help. It is better for her, overall and in the long run, to have to work her stuff *and* sometimes the family's, than to learn the technology of mentally directing herself away from expressing or given the tools of denial for yet another generation of emotional withholders.

Sometimes parents become distressed because their children are distressed, and with loving intent, would like to help them "stop feeling bad" by helping them to stop expressing as soon as possible. But once we engage on this path, we soon realize it feels worse to the kids to be forced to hold it in or otherwise dissuaded or distracted from letting it out. Expressing is not always "pleasant" for the child, but it is crucial for parents who are exploring new ways such as these to really look at the choice to allow or dissuade, to notice which is really the more unpleasant path for your child, and you, in the long run.

Bestowing The Blessing of Free Expressing

As parents we can, with awareness and application of tools that can work, minimize the amount of recovery our kids as future healing adults will have to do by allowing them spontaneous sound expression while still young. Kids need role models...and yet, kids themselves can be the model if they are allowed to be, in a sort of radical "and this little child shall lead" approach. If allowed, she can let her own emotions lead her. A child does not really always need an adult to model expression for them (though it absolutely helps when a parent is also involved in expression healing), when the natural course is allowed and given acceptance. Emotional intelligence has not been tested too often, except by those of us who have put in enough time and deeds at this point.

When first presented with the path of Healing and Dealing, most of us do not know that we will not just become raving lunatics at nearly all times and forever be having to run off to some makeshift scream room in the middle of dinner at a restaurant. Not that we will not get triggered in a restaurant; we will, and sometimes, until societal permission broadens, we will have to "hold it", like a bowel movement without an available toilet, until safe space becomes available. Finding safe space to express as soon as reasonably possible *is* important.

Encouraging Children's Emotional Understanding

Sometimes a child may know why she is angry after the anger has expressed and subsided. She may or may not be able to articulate it, and even if she can, she may not want to articulate it to her parents. There is no need to force the child. This way she can learn how to trust her own guidance and inner true understandings that she will undoubtedly receive from the aftermath of her expressing.

That said, there is nothing wrong with prompting them or asking them, maybe just after or after some time has passed, what they think they are really mad at. Waiting until after the release and perhaps after some time has passed can be best, so the child is not rushed into the word level prematurely. If it is just the surface thing that they say they were mad at, take that at face value, while suspecting they might find out more later.

Ask questions of your child to get information; go easy on inserting your own beliefs or speculations as understandings to give them for why they were angry. If you feel you really have some kind of intuition on it, decide in the moment -- and I would still suggest asking them if your insight feels true to them. Do not just tell them your intuition and then declare that that is why they were angry, because they may feel their inner wisdom usurped by such an approach.

After a child's expressions, encourage them to seek clues to find out what they think they were really mad about; perhaps they might be actually more sad or scared than mad, really, underneath it all (some emotions mask or "protect" the deeper, more vulnerable ones hiding beneath). I would not be surprised if there were a lot of tears that come during or after the rage. This is very common and something we all do -- mask grief and hurt with a layering of rage or mask anger with a layer of tears. All combinations therein are possible. We do this top-layer emotional presenting because most of us can and do "get away" with acting out the acceptable emotion in all the traditional ways. Our emotional body figures that it's going to get some airtime in one way or another, even if getting this airtime manifests in a way that does not really heal.

It is crucial to remember that the emotional body does not follow the same linear rules of decision making as the mental body; in some ways one might say they are from different planets. Once the rage is allowed to flow more deeply, the tears may not be far behind. Alternatively, fear may also be just under the presenting rage.

Layers of Seriously Repressed Emotion Surfacing

Allowing your child to begin to express after years of casually repressing their expression can reveal a potential scenario that contains a caution, something to look for if it happens, and yet, to not misinterpret as a "medical emergency" or something to take drastic action about. That is, once your child is allowed to peel layers back with her expressing, the child may or may not come upon some layers of emotion that would really love to express and yet, are so constricted with past internal and external pressuring that they may look very extreme, such as red-faced breathing difficulties.

What might happen in that kind potential scenario is that the child hits a gap within themselves where they have so programmed themselves/been programmed to not cry that they are holding back with all their might there, and need help at that point to let go. It would feel, perhaps, like a survival issue to them: "If I don't hold back my tears now, I will be hit! I will be hurt! I will have my face yelled in from up close by a very big person! I won't survive! I must hold back! But I can't hold back! ARGGGGGGG!!!"

None of this is mental, but it is in there for some people nonetheless, at the emotional belief level. This is where physical contact, holding the child and verbally encouraging them to cry if they need to could help them let go and cry and let out the possibly strangled-sounding sounds that have been held back so long, start breathing again, and recover that nearly asphyxiated part of them hiding within.

I realize this is potentially a very scary picture I am painting, and yet, since many parents are not doing this work themselves, it is important to spell out such a possible occurrence in graphic detail so parents could have at least have one example of what the inner state of

224

a compressed emotional body is like when it starts to surface from the deep.

Emotional Piggybacking

Anger, or any kind of emotional expression can reflect an incredibly complex dynamic. This complexity is most confusing *before* expression has run its course. There can be all sorts of reasons and non-reasons and other old emotional charge piling onto the initial trigger in a kind of piggybacking. In other words, when one major feeling is given expression when triggered, others "jump on" that have been held back, previously denied, but are now finding an outlet. There is a lot of inner sorting out that needs to happen in the aftermath, when the integration phase of the trigger cycle is engaged.

This integration cycle is very important so we can understand why we were so triggered. What were the real reasons why I felt what I felt? Understanding the root cause of our triggers is a key, final component in healing our old, held emotion. In the end, the complex of all emotions expressed in such a piggyback nearly always transcends whatever the initial surface trigger and scenario was about. This phenomenon was also addressed earlier in Chapter 9 "Backlog of Emotional Charge".

This can manifest as your child's reaction seeming all out of proportion to the trigger. The child in this case has a "backlog of charge". Old emotions that perhaps have nothing to do with the frustration at hand are piggybacking on the current moment's outlet and finding an opportunity to express in sound, which is what emotions naturally do when not shut down, suppressed, threatened and controlled, or talked out of themselves. Sometimes the quantity of overall charge ready to express in the emotional body is simply too powerful and big to have been curtailed to date by the controls already attempted, internally (the child's own attempts to "be good" or follow orders that they internalize) or externally (past accumulation of parental attempts to stop expression).

The child has now got all this old rage (or whatever emotion) coming forward on top of the surface level frustration at hand. Expressing this rage is perfectly healthy and normal, so long as doing so is not acting out on someone. Expressing anger in sound only appears unhealthy because of our sick societal relationship with emotions.

Much of what we have discussed under the rubric of children's emotional cycles is *not* only applicable to children. The cycles and tendencies outlined in this chapter are just as often embodied by adults, who are merely children who have had a grown-up shell coalesce around them.

Parental Choices for Handling Their Child's Emotionality

For the parent, the choice is to coach children to let their emotions out responsibly when they rise, or to put up with the eventual and often chronic acting out of the same emotions that never find true release. Children and some adults act out more readily than others because their walls of denial are not as strong as others' are to resist the pressure of holding these reined in feelings. The acting out of emotions happens when there is no inner or outer acceptance of them.

When deep primal expression is not encouraged, the only influence exerted upon children to help them deal with their emotionality is helping them attempt to contain acting out behavior inevitably resulting from lack of free and deep expression. Anger management techniques are mainstream society's attempt at controlling the power of emotions. For the most part these techniques, when looked at closely, are merely tools to help people of any age deny better.

Techniques can only work to a point and never actually resolve the underlying issue(s) at root for the child (or adults too for that matter). An appropriate comparison is the mood-altering prescription pill meant to adjust brain chemistry and control emotion that way, or drugs to kill physical pain, neither of which address the root issue. Addressing the symptoms of deep pain while overlooking or minimizing emphasis on root cause is a bad habit traditional medicine and society at large have adopted. Symptomatic focus is a bypass and not the path of healing and dealing, although sometimes medication can be helpful, as a band-aid is necessary on a deep cut until it heals more fully. A band-aid "solution" of medication is thus a temporary fix to buy time until the resolve is mustered to deal with the underlying issues.

No set of controls can keep emotions down forever -- but controls can indeed warp emotions' expression in the meantime, and result in all sorts of unsavory acting out. It is often harder on the parent when a child is routinely being triggered and expressing it than it is on the child -- sometimes the parent wants to change their child's reaction, so the parent does not get so stirred themselves. Parents may hate an overabundance of noise, because, well, it was not so cool when *they* were growing up to be too noisy! On the other hand, too much loud expressing in the room, even "appropriate" emotional expression, may simply be hurtful to the ears of others in the room. Encouraging a child to go in another room to make a lot of noise, or to yell into a pillow can be a win-win.

If your child is having uncontrollable anger, terror or crying outbreaks, it is possible that "the universe", that which is happening around us and to us, may be signaling you as the parent personally, via the reflection from your child. I made the point earlier in the chapter that kids are a natural outlet for their parents' denials. I have introduced tools that can be used when you as a parent are triggered by your child's expression or action. With practice, applying these tools can yield helpful results.

The other reason for this suggestion about your own expression is because, more often than not, kids really do look to their parents for modeling, psychically, visually, and experientially, and if you are holding back your own old feelings while encouraging them, they may well see or feel that something is not quite right with this picture, and take any input you have into their process as just another form of control – "do as I say, not as I do."

If your children are moving and moving (I use the term "moving" in this context to indicate expressing emotionally) over months and you decide not to go ahead yourself, and nothing much changes for them, then you might reasonably conclude that maybe they are just reflecting your own stuff back to you, while moving very little of their own.

Timeouts for Parents

Karen, who had broached the subject of an infant's public expression, also shared the following: "I know I have anger issues. I have not been sure how to deal with it because it smolders just outside of view without "forest fire ignitions". I will just freak out at my family in words after the kids raise the anger density in the room with all the bickering, baiting, teasing, poking, and hitting. I can easily see that that activity is reflecting my "acting out inappropriately."

Karen could easily be in full "ignition" -- that is, triggered to the point of easily being able to express in wordless sound -- if she were to take a personal time out for herself in the midst of those moments. If she were to wait until "the perfect moment" she may miss the window, however, as many trigger "windows" can be fleeting. Sometimes I have found I can miss anger trigger opportunities if I do not take advantage of them right away. In some cases the trigger is gone even ten seconds later.

The moments when ignition is possible can move into awareness in a split second and out just as fast. With experience I have become better at recognizing and capitalizing on them. As detailed in the previous chapter, it can be extremely helpful for a parent, and indirectly, for the kids, if the parent can just turn heel and march off to the bedroom, saying over their shoulder if need be "I need a time out by myself, I will be out when I can".

I mentioned earlier that fluffy pillows are best for sound nullification. Instead of letting it act out per age-old patterns that merely pass the anger back and forth, such as turning verbal dragon fire on mate or kids, perhaps allow it a different kind of expression in your own 'safe room', using pillows if you are feeling private or safer with your sound masked. Allowing ignition to lead to full sound expression affords the emotional charge a real possibility for shift.

Releasing Beliefs About Parental Emotional Responses

Judgment release, as detailed in Part 3, is crucial for relieving the mind's constrictions on experiential potential and goes hand in hand with emotional expression. When you release judgments, release as many judgments/beliefs out loud to yourself, with as much meaningfulness and feeling in the words as you can muster. Examples:

"I now release the judgment that expressing my anger hurts my kids if I let it out"

"I forgive myself for having believed for so long that I just need to find a different way to react and then everything will be alright"

"I release the judgment that I must "keep it together" for my kids at all times, so as both to set a good example and not to frighten them."

"I forgive myself for having believed for so long that I need to compress my true expression and have a better attitude to be a 'loving' parent."

You should have no trouble letting one judgment release lead to the next. They show up in my mind one after another like a little daisy chain, sometimes; the next one arriving to consciousness on the tail of the one I just let go, or attempted to let go. Judgment release is an iterative process. Like any other process, judgment release can become more effective the more it is practiced.

In these instances, emotional expression and judgment release, together with calling for the light of love to fill you, can result in lasting changes for the whole family.

Chapter 33: Sacrifice and Selfishness

I am learning to only help others if I really feel like it. I know that is counter to what many people say is loving. I naturally want to give to others, and go there often, because it feels good. I just intend to do it when I really want to, and that is partly what re-integrating my true feelings in each moment is about. The process of re-integration increasingly includes an awareness of what I truly want in the moment, the ability to respond to that awareness, and a decrease in taking actions driven by old conceptual guilt-ridden beliefs. When guilt can be released via the emotional movement process, one learns that there is no right or wrong in determining how much help to give. True giving comes from desire to give, in the moment, not from guilt or belief.

My friend Nathalie mentioned that it took her many years to find a balance of giving and receiving because of her Catholic background, which espoused forgetting the self completely in favor of others. She found that she needed to learn to contain her energy for a period of time and not help or give very much during this time. She found that the more she released judgments (particularly where listening to her true feelings and taking care of herself first was selfish and not to be trusted), the more she built a foundation of trust within her being and the more giving and receiving returned to a healthy natural balance.

Judgments on Putting The Self First

There are many judgments against putting oneself first. In perhaps all societies, people on the whole do not tend to put themselves first much, and certainly not without being stigmatized. The very act of putting oneself first too often is harshly put down and written off as "selfish, irresponsible, self-absorbed and unloving." "Putting yourself first leads to chaos and nihilism" is another popular judgment. Rarely is anyone commended for following his or her own truth if self-firstness is a common personal practice. (I prefer the word "self-first" to selfish.)

The only sustainable way for a human being to give that does not produce backlash is to give from a full or at least filling cup, and from pure desire to do so, not from some belief that "it's the right and loving thing to do" by somebody else's standards. I love to give, and I am very good at it, but I can no longer easily or readily give from an empty or nearly empty cup. Giving from an empty cup can chronically sap the life force from a person, resulting in illness and even death if balance is not sought.

Societies have never tried nor condoned giving to oneself and loving oneself first, and taking care of oneself in order that one can take care of another. A functional society would have a repercussion-free environment for pursuing free will. Instead, because of emotional denial, guilt is king and everybody is prone to taking guilt-based actions, including giving when they go past their own limits in order to do so.

The Cycle of Giving and Receiving

Many words have been spilled about how it's much more loving to give than to receive. But how can one give if there is no one to graciously receive the gift? Receiving is every bit as important as giving, because one act is not possible without the other.

Guilt and cultural imprinting have let us know that it can be downright shameful to receive too often – one risks being labeled a "taker". Saying yes to a hand extended without a lot of fanfare is a natural skill that many of us were shunted away from as we grew up. A simple "yes, thank you" is all that is necessary in order to gracefully receive an offer that we'd like to receive.

Many of us were also taught not to need anything, so to turn away offered help of any kind has been seen as the right response. This response, when it is not real, stops the cycle of giving and receiving in its tracks. There needs to be an organic flow of light and love passed among us, and it doesn't have to be linear. In other words, because you give to me, it doesn't necessarily mean that I am in debt to you. It might be better in some cases if I "paid it forward", whatever "it" is, and help someone else when I can. Agreements can be flexible here.

We all need help from time to time, and learning how to acknowledge need, ask for help, receive help and face any emotions or judgments inherent in the process of asking can be a process.

A Free Society?

We in western culture live an illusion of freedom, but we are not really free. Due to having chronically denied our personal power, we are time slaves, economic slaves, slaves to rules and strictures. We are subject to inequities and enforced controls overseen by an external global power who has a very specific agenda to curtail freedom while repeating a mantra that it is protecting and preserving freedom instead.

At the collective level, this is the outer reflection of rules curtailing freedom to act as we see fit, originally caused by inner denial of free will. We often deny ourselves what we really feel like doing with many should's, frozen fears and judgments. After many generations of engaging in this pattern, we have negated our free will to do what we really feel like doing, to the point where our denial is "out there" placed firmly against us. Many of us appear victims to the "powers that be".

One way to start undoing this imbalance is to try allowing what we feel like doing and see what happens. At first, long-denied personal desires may rush forth and begin to act as selfishly (in the traditional sense) as judgments held against them say they would if allowed to be free. These judgments and intertwined emotions must be released for the desires to find eventual balance in their manifestations. True balance does not sacrifice personal desire and the self, nor does it override and abandon loved ones nearby who are dependent or need help. When we have had enough experience and triggered releases, fears and judgments around sacrifice and selfishness can disappear and stop fueling the macrocosmic reflection.

Sacrifice and selfishness are two extremes on a continuum, and neither pole is a balanced place. Continually giving to others from an empty cup will result in a crash and burn. Conversely, giving only to the Self can reflect a shrouded heart that does not let others in or allow a natural flow of energy toward others in our lives.

Sometimes selfishness, in its least appropriate guise, is a reaction from chronically not giving to the self or believing the self worthy. It is the result of not having given love to the places that need it most. An ongoing lack of self-love can boomerang into a desperate, grabby need for energy from outside, perhaps in forms such as attention, money, fame, services, and general help. When this pattern evolves and love and self-nurturing is present, a decrease in what is needed from outside the self can be noticed, and an overwhelming desire to share this love can come forth.

I AM a whole universe, contained within myself. I AM life. I desire life. My desires and my life force and essence are priceless. When I give to myself, I AM giving to the All by vibrating self-love across the psychic realms, across the hologram that we exist in.

Chapter 34: The Family Contract

My first awareness of a contract of any kind came to me as a child, in the form of the ubiquitous electronic presence in my life growing up -- the TV. "Lost In Space" was one of my favorite shows, and in one memorable episode ("The Trader"), a Mephistophelian rogue from another planet binds Dr. Smith to a contract. Smith and the space family Robinson are marooned on a desolate planet with little food, and Smith decides in his inimitable self-first way that he is going to trade spaceship fuel for food. Little does he know there is fine print attached to the Trader's contract, which Smith signs by imprinting his hand in the soft-clay surface of a box. Unbeknownst to the good doctor, this contract actually compels Smith not merely for delivery of getaway fuel from the lost planet, but also for his very life and soul essence. Smith has signed a deal with a devil.

In this chapter I purport that we also have signed a contract with our family just by unconsciously choosing to be born into it, and we are no more aware of what we have agreed to than Smith was.

Hallmarks of The Family Contract

During my first year after moving to British Columbia, a psychically attuned kinesiologist gave me a psychic reading. During the reading she spent a long time talking about the intense psychic family contract that I have been bound by at a subconscious level. Such family contracts are not uncommon, she informed me, and can be incredibly powerful and obligating.

The theme of The Contract varies across families who have them. Many, or even most families perhaps, have these subconscious contracts, though there are some families that are more chaotic to the point where a contract does not apply. Also referred to as "unwritten rules", family contracts vary in strength and enforcement depending on the family.

Some families are comprised of powerful and talented individuals with huge potential, both realized and latent, but unfortunately that power is often tied up in or bled off by strictured, structured energies that do not allow the co-existence of free choice and a flow of love without strings attached. Much love, personal power and latent greatness is tied up in The Contract itself instead of being manifest as the free flow of energy among the lives of individuals within the family.

Everybody in a family can feel or describe the presence of The Contract if they tune into it. The individuals within families are obviously all very closely connected psychically as well as physically / genetically, whether there is conscious awareness and acknowledgment of it or not.

Some examples of tenets within family contracts are: an agreement among members of the family to study and work hard, get ahead by finding and keeping an upwardly mobile but traditional job in a company or similar hierarchical organization, save for retirement, become as wealthy as possible, turn the bulk of energy and attention back into the family, sacrifice any personal dreams while having kids who, although allowed to have fun and playtime growing up, must never break the family mold once they come of age, including paying back the family for the sacrifices the family made for them.

Self-sacrifice is a hallmark of many classic family contracts. Many family contracts call for the current parenting generation to sacrifice for the next generation.

Family Contract Roles

Roles in families are often played out unconsciously, inexorably perpetuating The Contract. There is usually an "executor", a member of the family, a patriarch or matriarch, who models the tenets of The Contract while enforcing their necessity with a heavy hand upon others, either children or siblings. To balance the executor there must be one or more "black sheep" across the generations - the rebel, the iconoclast who attempts to break free of The Contract.

Within the family contract paradigm there are also "law-abiders" who do not necessarily prosper under or enjoy the rules, but believe they have no choice. The law abiders stay within the bounds of The Contract and make the best of them. Often in this subgroup there is significant unprocessed rage and hurt about their own childhood interaction with, and shutdown at the dictates of the family contract. In order to prevent old, unwanted emotions such as fear, anger or hurt being stirred too close to the surface, the law abiders participate in backing the executor in enforcing the shutdown energy inherent in The Contract. If, like the executor, they try to shut down the rebel energy in the family, they are outwardly mirroring the inner shutdown of the individuals involved.

There can also be a fourth subgroup, former "bad kids" who make a few inroads toward breaking The Contract. After some setbacks and consequences directly or indirectly meted out by the executor or law abiders, the "bad kids" fall eventually back into line, neither supporting outright rebellion nor adherence. In some cases, this group will deny the existence of The Contract.

Free Will And Obligation

The amount of success or failure of the rebel to free herself of the confines inherent in the family contract is in direct proportion to the amount of personal power she has relative to the family and the executor. Depending on the executor's relationship with the rebel, and each's ability to shift and change, at some point the executor must ask himself which is more important: The Contract and its unwritten rules and codes of behavior, or the free will of the rebel, and his or her love for the rebel?

On the other end of the polarity, the rebel must ask herself a similar question: which is more important, my free will or my obligation to the family? She must be willing to risk this sense of duty in order to remain true to herself and her heart's desire which allows her to break free of the bounds of The Contract.

A friend asks: "What about the love inherent in the rebel's family obligation? She has two pieces of love, one for family and one for free will. Where is the balance point and how does it move? Is there love under the guilt, or not? If there is not much else besides guilt, is acting on its urging caving in to pressure, or habit? Guilt has to be holding on to something...what is that? Is there free will within obligation?"

This is a very excellent series of questions and there are no pat answers I can give. If one does truly feel free and at free choice within the bounds of duty, then to me, duty is transformed into the love of giving. If it feels right to give to the family in a certain way and that is congruent with being true to oneself, then by all means, one's will to give can be followed.

This, however, is not my definition of obligation and duty to the family. Obligation means "you have to" regardless of whether you want to, or whether it is your truth to give that action or time or re-direction of your life's goals if they are not in alignment with the dictates of the family contract.

What the rebel in any given family is nearly always facing is the reality that her goals, dreams and right action for herself is not "what is usually done in this family". If they entered a family at birth who would support their free will choices, their choices would automatically be in alignment with the highest ideals of that family's executor, and freeing themselves from a family contract would probably be a null issue. Ultimately, if a rebel finds herself in a role of needing to break free from something, she has had a karmic history of denying herself on behalf of others in an imbalanced way, i.e. choices made in self-interest were not in balance with choices made to please or serve others.

The Contract needs to be acknowledged, experienced and felt, and finally seen for what it is in order for evolution to occur at all levels of family. To some degree it morphs and shifts through and among the generations, as each new family branch and member gets brought into the psychic mix through marriage or birth.

Family Types

There are also different species of "family" such as spiritual families, blood families, emotional families, ethnic families and so on. Contracts and norms exist within all these families. Any contract needs to be acknowledged, experienced and felt for its hidden power to be fully undenied by the participants.

Spiritual families are found among doctrines, particular healing paths or practices. Norms that have accreted over time in these families are like norms in any other type of family, and must be felt through by each individual in order to fully experience what is of service to their personal path and what is to be discarded. Contract breaking may be more subtle in such families, but it is still real.

Emotional families may be ad-hoc families consisting of friends who have bonded deeply over things such as mutual tragedy, addiction recovery, intentional communities or simple simpatico. Rebellion or adherence to unwritten contracts need to be conscious choices in each moment, in order for the family at hand to remain functional and growthful for each individual. Ethnic families also support codes of behavior, for better or worse, and also must be felt deeply in order to determine what is most useful for personal growth and self-realization.

Free Will Within Families

Loving family bonds were never intended to become rules of enforced behavior that hinder a given individual's free will to choose and act according to how that individual sees fit. Ideally, loss of love and inclusion should not have to be the price to pay for being true to oneself.

A free will action ideally harms none, while offering safe triggers. If the rebel makes a free will choice that challenges her family contract, then growth and evolution, including some form of death (not necessarily physical) is inevitable. Death in this instance can mean death of the current family structure, death of the definitions and "look" of one's previously-held place and reputation within the family, and possible death of active relationship between the rebel and certain members of her family.

Does such a potential death indicate a failure or loss? Not necessarily. Sometimes an old structure must fall in order for something new to take its place, take the space where the old and no longer useful structure had been. Grieving for the emotional experience of loss of the familiar, no matter how dysfunctional, may indeed be part of the process for all concerned who are in touch with their emotions.

Many family contract "executors" have not evolved much in their time within the family, for to be an executor means one sacrifices personal will for what obligation dictates, according to the contract. Without an active personal will, it is not possible for human beings to evolve outside the closed system of "what must happen". Our definition for personal will within Healing and Dealing includes one's ability to respond emotionally and thus able to flow with change. Executors have gotten stuck in frozen images of "what is right". In a closed system such as this, no role outlined in a family is internally or externally free to evolve within their own family contract.

If the executor's child attempts to break the family contract, it can feel to the executor like a rejection of their love and what they are offering, as though their entire worth is being undermined and called into question. The message is, "this is what it was for me, and has to be what it is for you, because if it's not it says something to me that I don't like."

The executor has supported the rebel all their lives within the contract's dictates, which can feel like a long-term investment to the executor. When the contract is declared null and void by the rebel, it may feel to the executor as though something wrong and unfair has happened. At this point, the executor is at a crossroads of choice; on one hand, he may choose to feel how everything really feels to him and dare question the validity of the family contract he has been tasked to and worked so hard to uphold. Otherwise, he may likely wall up against the rebel and deny any emotional response that may start to arise for him.

Everyone involved in the family contract is presented with a choice, for after all, we are each born into certain families because that is the situation wherein we have the greatest opportunity to learn about ourselves and our maximum potential for growth.

The Rebel Disowned

Ripping up the Contract is not everyone's path, and there will be a place for "law abiders" in families unless and until a more healed version of this picture emerges. As rebels break away from The Contract while still retaining every intention of remaining a part of the family, some executors attempt to artificially create a balance by cutting the rebel out of their heart. It is said that at this point a family matriarch or patriarch have "disowned" their daughter or son, excommunicating them from the circle of family. When conscious healing has not been involved, the consequence of breaking the family contract has often been, at the very least, a loss of love and estrangement of the rebel from the family. That loss is felt on many sides depending on how many members were intrinsically involved in enforcement or disobedience. The rebel and the executor are sure to be involved in this aggregate love loss.

Law abiders in a family, if they are in contact with the rebel, will often tell her that the executor loves her deep down. Yet that love is no longer accessible to the executor's conscious self. Love that was previously present is now denied. In the extreme, the love is now hidden under impacted, unprocessed anger or hurt which can over time accrete into hate. This can manifest in stony silences or grudges held as "punishment" from executor to rebel. However, love or real feelings denied may take other forms, such as indifference, blankness, pleadings from executor to rebel to return to the fold, emotional blackmail, threats, fears expressed as "fears for the rebel".

When the executor of the family contract excises the rebel from his heart for breaking The Contract, or when the rebel in turn excises the executor, they literally shove the love out of themselves. The love may exist, but out in the dark somewhere, unacknowledged, unowned and unfelt. When the love for his seeming polar opposite within the family is no longer accessible to the executor's or rebel's conscious heart and mind, the void that remains can morph into hatred, unless and until the issues underneath are deeply explored.

Psychic Effects of the Contract

Sometimes the rebel will feel the pull of The Contract, saying "come along now, you must do what is right". This can manifest as a feeling of hopelessness and inner powerlessness to resist, sometimes with overwhelming guilt. These feelings have the power to colour her whole day with shades of torpor and dullness, lack of desire to live, or feelings of "what's the use".

Core beliefs swim to the surface of the rebel's consciousness. As she releases them, she can feel energetic forms like spiky eggshells cracking off, and pockets of old emotional charge rising to the surface beneath them which she can then vibrate by allowing the sounds they want to make.

There is hell to pay for reneging on The Contract, and the rebel must heal the parts of herself still beholden to it. As she processes old feelings and faces her original judgments about how family life just 'is', she is in effect ripping and re-ripping up The Contract until it loses the power to control her actions or her life.

Voiding The Contract

A theoretically successful rebel voids all contracts, psychic and unspoken, including family, relational and societal ones that enforce compliance or remove love or privileges. She then draws in a replacement family, one that accepts her for who she is and acknowledges her as an evolving, changing being. To get to this point and not recreate the original family scenario complete with acrimony and loss of love, the rebel must feel the feelings and release the judgments that caused her to become originally ensnared in a contract which bound her freedom so tightly.

According to one classic version of the contract, the rebel needs to pay back to the executor and/or the family the time and energy that was originally sacrificed "for the children". When the rebel reneges on her side of that unspoken bargain, the consequences kick in. This pattern continues until The Contract is completely expunged from the rebel's life. This is done through exploring the depths of the old feelings and releasing the old charge all the way to the bottom of the psyche, to the point where the earliest familial imprints and judgments of how reality is supposed to be at home are changed not only consciously but subconsciously. You will know when subconscious transformation has occurred in this area only when enough time passes in the new family (which can be a re-jiggering of the old family, potentially) and evolution and joy are on a steady, upward track with no major reversals and loss of love and trust.

Along the way to this full healing, the former rebel can re-establish herself in a new and improved family situation that is in some fundamental way a substitute for the original family, unless the original family is also moved to stop following The Contract. The original family can never be truly replaced, but if all feelings of loss are balanced within the Self, certain needs that had gone unmet in the family of origin can be fulfilled and the sense of loss minimized.

It is also possible that family dynamics can shift and heal, that a rebel can return after some personal work to find a new environment waiting, and can lay down the mantle of "rebel". The former rebel may or may not be drawn to spend further time in the original family, but when interactions occur, she may be pleasantly surprised to notice that the dynamics have changed.

In the climactic scene of that "Lost In Space" episode, the barterer from hell shows up to claim his side of the bargain. He holds up The Contract facing Dr. Smith, the hand imprint glowing, and as Smith walks helplessly with his arm and hand outstretched towards the image of his hand imprinted in that contract, the Robinsons' cybernetic robot blasts The Contract right out of the trader's hand into space dust with a jolt of lightning.

If it could only be that easy outside the realms of fiction! Our real-life lightning jolt has to take a slower, more iterative form of releasing judgments aloud, and feeling the feelings that come up when we release those judgments. This allows understanding to seep in and old rejected parts of self to return and fill us in the places where the darkness of ignorance and self-denial had been.

The Global Family Contract: Government As Executor

On the macrocosmic level, oppressive governments reflect the unmoving rage inherent in The Contract, presenting as "obligation or consequences". The Contract appears to be in force today in the United States, in Britain, in Iraq, in Saudi Arabia, in Afghanistan, in Palestine and everywhere there is unrest, a civil rights cutback or civil disobedience. Massive societal change could be precipitated by an overt rendering and popular acknowledgment of the hidden "human family" contract.

How is this possible when we are just individuals and there is a mighty-seeming oligarchy or military in place to do the bidding of that oligarchy? As without, so within. It's really as simple as that. The microcosm has direct effect on the macrocosm, so it starts with us and our personal process of undoing our belief systems. It starts with us doing our emotional undenying work

If enough of us who have major latent personal power do this work, and keep going all the way down through the layers of denial, experience by experience, trigger by trigger, it is my feeling that the outer alignment of intimidating form positioned against us will be retrieved and balanced within. The more this happens, the more this power, formerly denied but now magnetized back to the self, will look and act very differently than when it was split off away from us in a state of denial "out there", where it had been coalescing into fuel for military power and their masters, the forces who wish to control and subject. These forces who control and subject are showing us how we have controlled and subjected our very own personal wills. There is a correlation more direct here than you might at first realize.

In other words, as we heal and deal, our retrieved personal power is the very same denied energy that used to empower the very same power used against us. "They" literally have no more power than what we have given them, unconsciously, through denying our emotional power, which in fact comprises our personal power in large part.

The Universal Family Contract

Life, and Creation, is holographic. From within the dimension of time and its sequential nature, we humans act out Father's and Mother's and Child's ancient, time-before-time patterns, until we apply some of the steps suggested in this book for healing the patterns that have been acting out in everybody.

We, in our families, act out the pattern of Our First Parents as it has passed down the Family Tree to us. The executor of The Universal Family Contract is the force of denied rage (also fueled by underlying denied terror and grief), appearing in the role of the entrenched, angry, wrathful First Testament God that must be appeased, or the destruction of everything might just happen. All must live according to His rules and mandates and woe to them that stir the mighty wrath of God by "breaking the law". "His" needing to be in control is a metaphor for all of us. We fear, as He did, what bad things might happen if we lose control of our emotions.

The Healed Family

Let's speculate on what a healed family that has ripped up or balanced the need for a contract might look like. Such a family represents the groundedness, comfort and security that few families on Earth have manifested to date, if any.

The honoring and respect for free will would be at the heart of such a family, for starters. A family-wide willingness to allow the former rebel of the family to lead by example would be present. What might that look like? It could appear as though members of the family formerly in the vanguard of support for the family contract are observing how the rebel allows her will to lead her. They learn about the state of their own emotional bodies/desire bodies/wills by taking in what the prodigal daughter (or son, of course) is embodying. Her moves for herself may or may not be moves the others would make at first, but the more her other family members absorb how she feels about herself now, and how those feelings of supreme self-acceptance radiate from her, the more they wish, in their heart of hearts, to know her secret for themselves. They have begun to take steps toward freeing their own wills from slavery and allegiance to doctrine, norms and "a right way to be".

As individuals such as those involved in Healing and Dealing free themselves and their own wills, that freedom naturally begins to positively impact small groups of individuals such as families, which then ripple out to communities, countries, and ultimately, our world.

Chapter 35: The Art of Loving Touch

Every mammal needs loving touch or it cannot thrive. We watch cats, dogs and horses nuzzling and licking each other, curling up together, and we feel warm'n'fuzzy. How about two humans lovingly nuzzling each other... in plain view... in a non-sexual friendship? Well! Witnessing that, sometimes we feel a bit queasy and uneasy.

Notice the strictures around human beings touching each other, and it is no wonder so many of us are touch-starved, even in committed relationships. It is not "okay" for non-mated friends to walk arm in arm down the street in western hemisphere communities, especially same-sex friends. Stroking a friend lovingly is not acceptable, even in private (unless the friends are in sexual relationship). A cross-gendered pair of friends are not encouraged to touch each other without a sexual agenda; moreover, we tend to presume such an agenda. These possibilities of loving human interaction are not taught in school, seen on TV or appropriately modeled by many parents or adults.

Touch or Violence

Societal morality has steered us away from healthy, loving, needful touch. War is in part caused by people who did not get touched enough as babies and children, who grow up to be adults continuing to receive little or no loving touch, and who act out that denial of touch by hitting, striking, shooting or bombing "the enemy". Ever notice how much easier it is to fight with a loved one when you are standing at a distance? If we are touching, attack comes much less easily.

The idea of separation is encoded into our very DNA. Many of us seek to restore a sense of oneness with all people, but the road towards seeing everyone else as "like me" rather than "different than me" is long, because we are dealing with genetic imprinting, which is reversible only after significant healing and dealing. Loving touch (even from oneself) that does not include intent to sexually arouse "feeds" body a crucial nutrient, and helps adults heal from the wounds of separation and attack, including sexual violation.

Non-Sexual Touch, for Self and Other

If you do not have friends with whom you can share appropriate loving touch, you can give yourself healing touch in the bath, upon awakening, or before sleep. Lightly stroke and/or gently squeeze feet, legs, pelvis, arms, torso, face and hair. Slow movement deepens the experience. Avoid deliberately attempting sexual arousal. Notice distracting thoughts that arise, without giving them too much attention, release any judgments you notice, and return your attention to the sensation and your breath. If any emotions swim up, feel and express them as fully as possible; these come with the territory. Many bodies have a lot of touch-starved years to recover from.

If you do have a friend, healing partner, lover or "touch group" to try this with, set a clear verbal intention in advance to revere and honour one another. This will help build trust and depth. With backs supported, sit facing each other on the floor, set a rough time limit, and take turns touching and stroking, moving slowly and respectfully down the body. Really breathe in the offering from your partner (most of us find receiving more challenging than giving). Avoid simply massaging, and see if you can take the risk of gentle, stroking touch.

Safe Touch for Young Children

If you have children, especially newborns and toddlers under a year old, or are about to have children, I highly recommend "contact parenting" for as many months into your child's life as possible. Jean Liedloff's "The Continuum Concept" and Ashley Montague's "Touching" are must-reads regarding the health and wellness benefits of constant levels of loving touch for very young children.

Chapter 36: Sexual Wounding

Within nearly every adult human lies the ability to bond and join with another adult at the deepest possible levels through sexual union. It is this ideal that keeps many of us searching for the perfect coupling to bring us the bliss we have heard about, that we dream is possible, and that we even fleetingly achieved one time, one night, years ago with somebody who is not even around anymore. True magic and power, the ultimate creative rocket fuel, is inherent in our sexuality, but in many of us it sure does not feel that way.

Some of us feel sexually depressed, ho-hum or downright averse to sexual interaction. On the other end of the continuum lie those of us intensively driven to attain this bliss, scrambling past one lackluster or okayish orgasm after another in a desperate urge to finally find "it", never stopping to feel the emotional backlog accrued along the way.

Two Patterns of Wounding

Two main patterns (with variations) of adult sexual wounding can be identified. Firstly, having sex when we do not really feel like it, caving to either internal or external pressure. Secondly, moving too rapidly into sex and, once engaged, towards orgasm. "Too rapidly" means suppressing the desire to take one's time, or succumbing to old habits of impatience or need for the orgasmic jolt (this is different from the oneness of union alluded to earlier).

The main agents of wounding involved here are sexual guilt ("I have been saying no a lot, I should give my partner a 'yes' this time", or "I don't want to hurt him/her"), sexual terror ("I don't DARE say no again", or "I'm afraid to slow him/her down, I'm afraid of their anger, I'm afraid of the backlash"), and sexual rage ("aren't you finished YET?!", or "c'mon c'mon it's going to be so good, let's keep GOING...what's wrong?! What do you mean, you want to stop?", or bodily pounding, acting out a desire to dominate, etc.). Though by no means an exclusive listing, these are some of the words associated with emotions that arise from a lack of inner and inter alignment with acting on sexual feelings.

To create space for oneness, we must clear out what keeps us divided from ourselves and each other. We cannot just go directly to feeling sexually patient by deciding so; we must really be there. When triggered before, during, or after sex, feeling and expressing these old, formerly-denied feelings can help, in all the ways previously described. If you can dare to stop and feel, notice how hard it is to stop! This is how strong our sexual conditioning is. Pursuing and wanting yummy sexual feelings is not wrong, but the backlog must be addressed whenever stirred, or else the yummies get achieved with a potentially harsh price that will be collected on sooner or later. If you go past yourself or your partner, subtly or overtly, this harsh price could come up again, likely stronger next time, in ways you can't suppress, harsher than it would have been if you had paid attention the previous time.

For example, let's say during foreplay I subtly pressure my girlfriend into going past her hesitation to have intercourse. She succumbs to my pressure, we have sex, and it's pretty good, but the orgasm is so-so and afterward, we can each tell there is something not quite right, something we likely ignored at a certain key moment. When I do the same thing again the next time we are engaged in lovemaking, she decides in the aftermath that she needs a break from the relationship, because her needs do not feel honored. This is one example of a harsh reflection that may never have arisen if I had just proceeded more slowly the previous time and not pushed through a 'no' from my partner.

Staying Present and Moving Slowly

To truly bond sexually with another means having as much (ideally all) of ourselves present. Being goal-oriented in order to "get to" feelings of oneness or union, or an orgasm is a good way to short-circuit the very states one is intending to achieve. Moving slowly, dropping all goals and coming into the present moment is a needful baseline when sexual or sensual arousal is present. Let the touch or warm connection with your partner that is happening right now be enough, if possible. Breathing deeply from the root chakra can help keep you in the moment, staying present with what is happening rather than what might happen. Following the current of where things are and where they organically and naturally want to move will grow the energy into a potentially magical state, if surrendered to in every moment without pressure or urgency.

If staying slow and present feels difficult or impossible, or if the feeling of urgency persists, suspect that your impatience is masking some judgments that are keeping anger or fear locked below the surface. Conversely, if a rise in sexual feelings or ardor leads to a freezing up inside or feelings of disassociation (i.e. leaving the body, either energetically or into random thoughts), suspect sexual terror, old feelings of hurt or unresolved feelings from prior sexual trauma lurking underneath. These feelings are ideally expressed in sound or body movement on the spot, if you and your partner can co-create space for them to exist.

Sexual growth means paying attention to everything we are feeling once sexual feelings come into our space. A healing and dealing approach calls upon us to "stop the train" and drop into the feelings so no part of us feels "gone past", or ignored. To go past parts of ourselves that are slower or "aren't sure about this" or are suddenly triggered, in order to "get to the yummies" creates more sexual denial. Sexual denial is one of the deepest and most trauma- filled states of denial on the planet, so our in-the-moment attention and dedication to our healing process is absolutely paramount here. We each need to do our part to undo this vast, collective traumatic sexual dysfunctionality we each have participated in. Every opportunity for spontaneous healing in this arena is golden.

The mojo can return if no steps or feelings are skipped, and any judgments that sexual interaction has to unfold according to a certain pattern or progression can be released as well. All judgments arising as a result of encountering something unexpected need release.

Sex for Pleasure *and* Healing

If your partner needs to cry during or after sex, encourage that. This clearing is absolutely necessary and does not reflect how well you "performed". These tears probably have nothing to do with you, other than the help you gave your partner with your very presence so s/he could open deeply enough to fully feel him or herself.

This crying could be about many things. The person may be feeling sad that the sex is never how s/he dreamed it could be. It could mean that s/he was reminded of his or her trauma, and sex has opened the door to these feelings. S/he may feel a tearful relief that things are so much more loving now than they've been in the past, and s/he's never felt so loved. And many more permutations and possibilities exist for why crying is happening after sex.

As with all feelings being expressed by yourself or someone close to you in the space, allow the feelings to completely finish expressing and subside before internally or externally inquiring what it's about. Asking about the source of the feelings during expression has a strong tendency to short-circuit the expression. In doing so, you or the other person has to lift into mind, and as a result the will/emotional body loses the focus and 100% attention she needs to express herself.

The more deliberately we can engage our sexuality, the more likely it is that we will feel ourselves fully as we go along, and not deny our feelings. Sexual interaction is not only for pleasure and union, it is also a crucible for the deepest and most needed healing and dealing possible.

Sex with a Survivor

What happens when we find ourselves partnered with a survivor of sexual abuse? Having been in that role myself, I find that the pattern seems to be that the focus on pleasure and eventual movement toward true union is only approached by way of much time spent in the healing crucible. In other words, by dint of having a strong healing focus and partnering with someone who is a sexual abuse survivor, more often than not my partner's abuse memories are triggered by any sexual activity. We give these moments center stage, knowing we can't find union without dealing with these triggers right in the moment.

For readability's sake, in the following discussion I am going to use feminine pronouns 'she' and 'her' to indicate the survivor, and 'he' and 'his' for the partner, with an understanding that in many couples the genders are reversed, or one gender's pronoun is not applicable.

There are some key points for partners of survivors to take in deeply. The first is that the survivor has been violated in the deepest point in her being, often more than once, and is likely at some point during any given sexual interaction to be triggered into a physical or emotional memory, even if she has already done a lot of recovery work. Because sexual violation touches the core of the individual, the recovery can last a lifetime. This reality does not preclude loving and joyful sex, but can include ongoing triggers that arise across time.

Safety defuses triggers. Safety also can paradoxically heighten triggers, because if they're unresolved and lurking, they finally feel safe to come up and out. Whenever conditions manifest that give the survivor a strong sense of safety within the parameters of the relationship as a whole, sexual triggers sometimes do not even occur at all. A healthy sexual relationship can then be experienced outside the overwhelming impact of triggers. Although a survivor may still be in active recovery, within the boundaries of safety non-triggered sexual relations with a survivor are completely achievable. Safety is not a component of sexual abuse. Therefore, "safe sex" – literally – is not associated with memories of abusive sex. But, the two arenas can overlap spontaneously and without obvious, linear logic. Be sure not to subtly wrong-make a survivor for having memories triggered by your safe sex. It is most often not something you "did" to her to trigger the memory.

Secondly, the partner's natural sexual desire in and of itself can also serve as a memory trigger for the survivor. His desire coupled with a feeling in the survivor that she is pressuring herself or feeling pressured to go past her reluctance can possibly result in her partner "wearing the face" of her abuser, in an emotional or visceral sense.

Survivors are hypersensitive to the slightest presence of sexual need or hunger in anyone coming on to them. This includes anyone, anywhere, anytime and is not limited to either the conscious or unconscious natural libido of another. In other words, one does not have to engage a sexual "suggestion" for a survivor to be sensitive to that energy. Another's sexual desire or intent may feel predatory in nature to a sexual abuse survivor, thus triggering alarms of warning. You don't have to be a survivor to glean predatory energy, but a sexual abuse survivor may have heightened sensitivity. Sex has been used as a weapon and survivors are suspicious that even a healthy libido denotes an ill-intended sexual agenda.

The Various Forms of 'No'

The most important word for the survivor and her partner is 'no'. No can be said gracefully and discreetly, either vocally or through the silence of body language. The lack of an overt, loud, distinct, undeniable or even aggressively asserted "no" does not negate the "no" itself. No means no, period. "Maybe," "I'm not sure," and ambiguity of any kind, including nonverbal/physical or energetic cues also means no in this context. A survivor's "no," acknowledged and acted upon by her partner contributes greatly to a sense of safety within the relationship.

For the most healing result, the partner of a survivor needs to back off sexual advance or interaction immediately upon hearing the word or even the intimation that the original reception to sex has shifted for the survivor. Anything else, such as her partner's ignoring or negotiating with the survivor's desire to stop, or his delaying stoppage, results in a reconditioning of the old wound.

The upside of the partner's impeccability is that the destroyed trust in the core wound of the survivor can rebuild more quickly if she can learn to trust that her 'no' has power. This is the healing recipe; the empowerment of the survivor which only the survivor can truly negotiate but which the partner can support. This is a necessary stage towards complete recovery for the survivor so that loving and fulfilling sexuality can manifest as the norm. The partner can help the survivor, and in turn, himself by assisting the potential of this manifestation by being impeccable in respecting his partner's limits of the moment.

Consent and requests to try something sexually or to go further also enhance the safe space for everyone, not just survivors of abuse. People who are asked for consent are affirmed in the reality that they have choice as to where, or whether, to proceed. This is especially important with regards to people whose 'no' previously did not have power to change their outcome. When in doubt, get consent before proceeding.

A survivor of sexual abuse who has an authentic yes to proceeding sexually in the moment with her lover can, in an ideal scenario, understand that her 'yes' can turn into a 'no' at any moment and that it will be honored. Similarly, an authentic yes can emerge from a time of non-consent, if the no was honored. The safety inherent in that flexibility, if it exists, makes her 'yes' every bit as important as her 'no'.

Mutual Responsibility

The onus is ultimately on the survivor for owning and managing their sexual triggers, yet an equal onus is on the partner for their triggers in response to the survivor's triggers and behaviors regarding their sexual relationship. A key note for partners of sexual abuse survivors is paying attention to the reflection being offered by the survivor. The underlying question for partners to ask themselves is, "Why have I attracted a partner who is a survivor of sexual abuse?"

The partner will be tested in his ability to safely and appropriately express feelings of angry frustration, grief, hurt or terror and judgments that "it will always be like this", "I don't think I can stand being thwarted like this forever", etc. It can be terrifying for the survivor to experience her partner expressing or even having such feelings, but this dynamic seems quite necessary for healing to occur on both sides of the equation. It is crucial that the emotions here are handled responsibly, which can be a difficult task. Allowing wordless sound as soon as you can redirect yourself from any blaming expression towards purely unwinding the emotions and releasing the judgments attached to them is what is called for here. Blaming the other is often a stepping stone that we can intend to walk through as soon as we can, after which it is necessary to then completely own the emotions rising up for healing.

Closing the sexual gap between lovers means expressing and being honest and upfront with feelings on both sides, no matter what those feelings involve. Because of the depth of the issue at hand, this process can be akin to handling dynamite or nuclear waste safely, yet it must be done, no matter how many missteps, for overall evolution to occur in this most sensitive of relational arenas.

Undoing Rape Culture

Any sexual dark-side trigger is worth taking advantage of. The participants in a given world drama (think Kavanaugh, Cosby, Ghomeshi, Weinstein) are simply occupiers of the spotlight du jour, by no means the first, and they shall not be the last to stand off on this issue.

For most of us who don't personally know the people involved, it's not about them, at the end of the day. It's about what it brings up in us. It's about what it brings up in women who get thrown into all of the horrific memories of being sexually overridden, in subtle to major ways across the continuum, and how they are eloquently and passionately sharing their pain in response to a given outward drama. It's about what it brings up in me, as a man. Guilt, shame, fears about myself and what I don't know about in my subconscious, what it means when I furiously deny. Some questions I ask myself are, how do I collude? Who is my inner accused abuser and what does he look like?

How about when I doth protest too much, in a kneejerk way that is covering up my feared responsibility, to a woman, any woman in my past or present who points out where she felt violated by me? Even if the violation wasn't a big-ticket item like rape. Am I denying doubt, guilt or shame? In most cases, if not all, I think so.

Or maybe I forgot, or wasn't in my right mind. Denial is tricky and we're so good at it we can black out either via drugs, alcohol or simple refusal to notice or accept. That's when my defense is at its most intense, when I'm sure I'm right. "I don't remember" is a different animal than "I didn't do that!!!!", because when the latter is shouted enragedly, I probably have something I'm hiding.

Here is what I would say to you, now, to any woman I may have knowingly or unknowingly sexually or energetically violated at any level of the spectrum, in my past, present or future, from my heart and my place of ownership. May this also go out to any woman who has never received ownership and receivership from her abuser/violator, and where it wouldn't hurt to hear it from a man, this is also to you -

I believe you. I'm sorry. You don't ever deserve to be overpowered or gone past sexually. When I went past you, I couldn't stop myself. I was not in control, and I am ashamed of my lack of appropriate control. Some part of me knew what I was doing and didn't step up or couldn't step up to stop myself. I open to receive your feelings about this, about what you experienced me doing. I admit I need your help and your reflections, else I can't see exactly where, when and how I am being unloving. At the same time I go past you, I am going past myself.

I commit and intend, again, to listen, receive and own my dark sexual actings-out and the guilt and shame inherent in those moments. If I can, I commit and intend to stand up with women to say no to sexual molestation and overpowering. I commit to and intend listening to and respecting the limits and boundaries of my own inner feminine, my own 'no', my own intuition.

It is a male problem when women suffer sexual assault, not just "their" problem and survival issue. It's every bit a male problem when we men "deny until we die", to quote a university age man accused of multiple sexual assaults. It's about the overarching male-female dynamic, sexually, which every pubescent human is part of. As nearly every woman has gotten sexually overridden in some way, large or small or in-between, likewise nearly every man has involvement, be that involvement ever so subtle or long ago. That includes me, and perhaps any male reading this.

If the pot gets stirred, then it needs to get stirred, or it wouldn't be happening. Let the triggers fly, let the stories be told when and where and to whom there is enough feeling of safety. We need it to go back and forth until it is all cleared up.

It's time for myself and my brothers to step up and take responsibility for our side of things, to question and try to stop engaging the old habits. It's time to listen to women's #metoo stories and acknowledge, even if only to ourselves, that yeah, I did something like that before, I've acted out on that continuum.

I feel compassion for women, because I can't know what their journey is like, I can only imagine it. It sounds horrifying, and I love them enough to stand up and say I HEAR YOU. What my gender has done is egregious and I hate it. I will always stand with you around what happened to you.

Resisting and Receiving Female Outrage

"I hate generalizations, that's not fair, what about all the good men." I hear this phrase from both men and women when presented with what I brought forward in the previous segment.

When I've said stuff like this in the past, and I have been there, I could look under the covers of my outrage and notice what I was really feeling was upset that I wasn't trusted, unlike all those other bad dudes, as I was "a good man" and I knew that about myself. I knew other solid men. WE wouldn't do such things, c'mon!

In my best moments, I am okay with a woman not trusting me...those are her feelings, and may or may not say anything about my own trustworthiness. Considering the statistics and most of their herstory, women have every right to express mistrust, fear, rage, hurt about what has happened to them, how they and their sisters have been violated on the continuum of subtle to heavily by men.

Deep in the mix, often hidden and well defended from being felt/experienced in our male psyche is old denied shame. Shame from the mistakes we made in the sexual arena that were never put quite right, or left unaddressed. Shame that we participated in that continuum at all, one time, five times, ten times, be they all "subtle" pressuring or more.

I feel our denied shame gets stirred underneath it all when we men make statements like that; that we fear we might be as bad as the lack of trust from a woman seems to be saying we are. Maybe we have done things we are ashamed of, but have long since "denounced" those actions and evolved. That's great, and, we *still* might have hidden shame and/or guilt that drives us to say 'hey what about all the good men'. Ask many women and they'll often resignedly hashtag #notallmen when confronted about whether they really think there aren't good, respectful men out there. If men need to protest about women speaking out, I have learned that that is a signal that they need to look at this denied stuff. We had a LOT of programming that made it okay to violate a woman's boundaries, push the envelope in the name of "passion" and an unearned sense of entitlement.

It makes sense that most if not all of us have acted out at some point. By definition that puts some guilt or shame into the mix. It's time to get real and process this stuff out with those whom we men trust, get it off our chest and out of the dark through brave ownership, and support women speaking out and speaking up.

Stand

Sexual harassment of women

at any level
is not okay with me.
I take responsibility
for the subtle ways
I control and
overpower she
With my voice,
with my insistence,
with my (unconscious) choice,
with my resistance
with my silence

My persistence
to learn
to listen
to yearn
with women
for respect
for their bodies
their boundaries
to expect
they might be hurt
inside from my kind
I forgive my ignorance
Where I'm blind
I try again
Not "for you"
But for Us
We can heal these crimes
One responsibility-taking man
At a time.

Your safety is paramount
With you I stand
To surmount
The habits
The programming
Yeah I fuck up
I've lost count

of the times
When I didn't
let you finish
Didn't take you seriously
Acted imperiously
Didn't remember
Acted insidiously

I intend to hear
I intend to listen
To honour and
Face my fear
Of feeling guilt
or inferiority
Won't push it out
Onto her anymore
No, she def
Shouldn't take it
Anymore
I will hear your story
I will open to your hurt
Your rage, your fear
Your mistrust
Let's be men
Who won't say
"This has already
been discussed".

Abuse,
A continuum
Power over
Starts small
Call it out
Call a spade
A spade
It's Unacceptable!
And a poor trade
For the love she gives
For the life she lives

To heal herself
I support you
Except when I
Make a fool
of myself.

When a woman
Points out where
We men are offtrack
We need to listen
Not shove back
Not rise up bigger
Not talk smack
Not get louder
Or deny her trigger

I am he for she
Except when I
Forget and remain
Part of the problem.
I stand with men
Who stand with me
And stand for her
Not 'them' but 'we'
If it's her problem
It's my problem
We don't win
If she doesn't
And our society
Needs grow up
To be truly free.

Chapter 37: You Can't Always Get What You Want

There is a wonderful organization based in Northern California called the Human Awareness Institute. HAI taught me a formula for interpersonal manifestation that I am still working on fully implementing in my life since I first heard it over twenty years ago. HAI outlines three steps reflecting Mick Jagger's punch line to this chapter's title: trying sometimes gets you what you need.

1) Ask for 100% of what you want, 100% of the time;
2) Be willing to hear 'no'
3) Negotiate for a win-win.

In my exploration of this map to fulfillment, I have found there are additional steps that are not apparent amidst the formula's surface simplicity. I have expanded the list of steps, to where the formula now looks like this:

Step 0) Take the time to discover exactly what you want.
Step 0a) Ascertain that what you want is available now
Step 0b) Beware of what you don't want.
Step 0c) Process as many feelings as possible around having what you want.
Step 1) Ask for 100% of what you want, 100% of the time
Step 1a) Ask directly

Step 1b) Find/process your rage, fear and hurt around the possibility of hearing 'no'.
Step 2) Be willing to hear 'no'
Step 3) Negotiate for a win-win.
Step 3a) Process feelings if a win-win cannot be found at the end of negotiation.

This process has been created in the context of asking for something from someone else. Asking the universe for something can also involve a similar process. However, the intent of the "formula" given by HAI was in the context of asking another person for something.

Below is some explication of the additional steps:

Step 0) Take the time to discover exactly what you want. Does the person you are approaching have what you really want? We all have significant inherent power and magic to manifest. However, we often manifest what we think we want, which turns out to not be what we really wanted, because we have not taken the time to get to know our desire of the moment. We feel a desire arise, and then some other part of us instantly interprets what that is, and another part is off and running to get it. Whoa, Nelly!

Knowing whether what you desire is a deep need or not is important as well in this regard. Is what I want optional, something I can do without? Or is it a core need, something I feel I must have, and therefore am willing to go through all the steps in order to find some form of it?

Step 0a) Ascertain that what you want is available now

If it's not available, it's wrong time to ask. If it's going to be available in the future, or you perceive that it is, it may be prudent to wait until that availability becomes obvious – because what if your desire changes in the meantime?

Step 0b) Beware of what you don't want.
How many times does our wish begin like this: "I don't want..." Some examples:

→ I don't want to have another fight with him.
→ I don't want to have to wait in a long lineup.
→ I don't want to face these emotions.
→ I don't want to drive all that way.

This kind of "negative" wish can be made to someone else or simply to the universe. Often what I am really saying is, "I fear this thing happening," which is powered by an underlying judgment, "If it happens it will be bad and I won't like it."

Creating from unexamined or unprocessed fear, anger and judgments that are underneath every "I don't want" can give me what I fear. If I process the fear and release the judgments involved, I can discover what it is I am really afraid of. Noticing that there is always an "I want" behind the old "I don't want", and then asking for what I want can then put me back on track to manifesting positively and in accordance with true desire. Thus, re-workings of the examples above might look like this:

→ I want to have friendly, cooperative interactions with him
→ I want to spend as little time in line as possible
→ I want to feel good
→ I want someone else to drive, or I want to feel engaged and stimulated during my trip, or, I want the necessity of having to drive all that way eliminated.

"What I don't want" is a step along the way to finding what I do want. Most often the healing and dealing release of emotions and judgments around what I don't want clears the pathway to what I want.

Step 0c) Process as many feelings as possible around having what you want (e.g. worthiness issues, judgments against the possibility of success, fear of asking). A successful manifestation of truest desire has the greatest possibility of occurring if emotional triggers can be allowed and expressed ahead of time.

Step 1a) Ask directly. Notice that it always feels better when you yourself are asked directly for something; there is no feeling of undercurrent expectations or subtle manipulation. Example of indirect approach: "I've been thinking I don't want to go alone to the dance." Direct: "Would you go to the dance with me?"

Step 1b) Find/process your rage, fear and hurt around the possibility of 'no'. Doing so will assist you in releasing any expectations and temptation to manipulate the person.

Fear of hearing 'no' can result in indirect asking, not asking, or asking for less than 100% of what you really want. This is a key in the original three-step formula. If you are not willing to hear 'no', it is probably the wrong time for asking at all, and more process time is required first.

Step 3a) Process feelings if a win-win cannot be found at the end of negotiation. If a win-win cannot be found, how can you get what you need? Feel the core of your need deeply, express all the feelings you can, then stay aware for new information from without or within. Find willingness to hang out in the uncertainty of unmanifested desire, holding a line of faith that something will shift the situation toward getting your deepest needs met. "But if you cry sometimes/you might find..."

Releasing the Attachment to Outcome

Emotions need to be processed before they can truly evolve and release the pent-up charge they've held from being denied. We can't just let go of them. But in the realm of mind, it's a whole different story. It's very important to let go of and release attachment to pictures of what the mind fantasizes and envisions that it wants. Notice that the thoughts happen, and let them go without chewing on or obsessing over them, if possible. If that doesn't feel possible, it is quite likely that emotions are available to be felt into in order to help ease obsession.

The will burns desire, a raw force used by the mind to go down a track toward a picture it thinks it wants. This is a habit that everyone participates in, and it can be evolved like anything else in the Self. Letting go of the way you think you want it, without releasing the desire itself is a new practice to be cultivated in order to heal the relationship between your mind (mental body) and your will (emotional body) regarding desire.

Mind has always gotten attached to outcome and how it looks. It gets stuck in previous experiences because it doesn't know anything else. Mind has a tendency to repeat habits or draw from past situations because that is all it knows. This limits the potential of manifesting what I truly want in an evolving and new way. The marriage between desire and intention involves letting go of judgments and beliefs around the *having* of the thing. Mind has been attached to having, as well as the goal of needing to have it *right now and in this way*, which doesn't leave space for right time. Intention holds the space for desire to happen naturally, without the will being overly steered and without being co-opted.

Sometimes "negotiating for the win-win", a la the HAI maxim, may involve trying too hard. Mind fulfilling desire's wants is not mind's right role. Compromise is also not what negotiating for the win-win means. Compromise is based on a core belief that there isn't enough to go around so we all can get only a percentage or a piece of what we want at the best of times. If I hold the intention that everyone gets what they want in right time and right form, compromise does not have to happen.

Releasing judgments about what I think I want is very important to the Self's attaining a sense of fulfillment that comes from manifestation in the moment, thanks to the divine desire within all of us. What I am really after is the *feeling* I wish to feel if I had what I desire, or what I think I desire.

Chapter 38: The Fulfillment Path

Everybody wants and needs outside support and encouragement to make changes toward a fulfilled life. Fulfillment in this context really means being on my path, doing what I came to do. Doing what I came to do means doing what feels good or perhaps at times ecstatic. When I do what my essence is here to do, life force flows naturally and serendipity becomes the norm.

We often carry past associations with the concept of 'fulfillment' that we might have taken in and taken on subconsciously. In that picture of fulfillment, we only will feel fulfilled when we finally arrive somewhere. Questioning and releasing the judgment that "I can't feel fulfillment on the journey, just at the destination" can be helpful. The path is really meant to be fulfillment itself, at least in potential, and it will *never end*. There is really no destination!

Healing and dealing leads to greater self-acceptance. As we practice the tenets described in this book, acceptance for our emotions, our emotional body, our inner divine will grows within. We begin to transform our perception of the path as something to be endured to an actual growing sense of fulfillment. Yet we haven't "gotten" anywhere. We are still always traveling, with mileposts to be celebrated and responded to all along the way. When movement and change is occurring and flow is happening, we are being fulfilled. When we are fulfilling ourselves, we have energy for life. We don't ever really stop somewhere and stay, statically fulfilled for all time.

Fulfillment *can* be of course found in the actualizing of one's goals. Fulfillment is also possible all along the road of experience that is never intended to come to a conclusion. It's available now, not someday, and we'll know it when we feel it. It can be felt in getting a strong head of steam and progress on creative projects, or making healing breakthroughs from past traumas and patterns that are affecting our present moments. It can be felt in finding a partner, changing career, attracting greater abundance of (fill in the blank) or moving to another place on the planet to which we're drawn, where it feels good. Fulfillment can be found in simpler manifestations such as finding a friend, or breathing fully and staying present in our bodies. At essence, fulfillment brings a love for the fact that we feel good, or at least better now, and are headed in a direction we like that is bringing joy to the experience. We are passing through a good place.

Working to Change

Healing and dealing can be hard work, some of the hardest work we will ever do. Fulfillment can sometimes seem a long way off when we are in the midst of transforming dark places. Often when we start to enact changes in our lives, we find ourselves faced with all manner of dissuasion from partners, friends, or family members. Outer resistance such as this reflects inner resistance to change and growth, judgments we have bought and internalized as "reality". They tell us we are not able to shift, it is too hard, too much work, don't have the time or talent, too much negativity in the space – the litany goes on.

In the absence of 100% validating, positive inside and outside support (nobody has this so far), we manifest or encounter psychic and/or physically manifested obstacles, reflecting in exact measure the relative strength of our inner barriers to fulfillment. Instead of moving forward, when we hit these obstacles we can get discouraged, feel "set back", slow down or stop when we hit them or feel hit by them. Any feelings of discouragement, or reactions that include slowing down or stopping are certainly not wrong responses or feelings to have – we may need more time to stop and feel our feeling response more deeply, and wait for our slower parts to catch up. They and other feelings have things to show and teach us, perhaps about what happened the last time momentum on our path started to rev up. How did we feel then, that we went past back then in our hunger to get to the destination as fast as possible? What happened to stop us? How did I feel about myself when I was thwarted before? A host of layered emotional response is possible to be discovered here.

The obstacles are inevitable; seeing them as part of the fulfillment path is important. They already existed inside us. If they were not there, we would already have manifested our lives in an exact match of our visions and heart's desires.

It's not wrong to stop and rest, and it's not wrong to feel waves of self-doubt either, or any other despairing feelings, including that one is "not doing the path right" (i.e. the voice of guilt). Noticing the stories that pop up in response helps us to see them for what they are - not truths, but perceptions in a difficult moment, colored darkly. Then we move feelings and judgments hopefully, we get understandings, we talk to friends, we wake up in a new day a day or three later, and we might well feel differently. But it's not wrong for the moment to feel like hell sometimes.

Getting the Help We Need

How to deal? We need help. Help takes many forms – supportive friends, partners, family members and colleagues who believe in us, encourage our healthy risks, receive or witness us when we vent, offer analysis and solutions when those possibilities are requested, and take responsibility for their own stirred emotional responses to what we are trying to do.

If this kind of help is not organically forthcoming, we need to seek it and ask for it from all corners of our support network, or elsewhere. Perhaps we seek it from our inner divine source, who is there for us and awaits our reaching out for help. This in itself is a challenge for many people, especially, but not limited to, men who were raised with do-it-yourself conditioning. The above forms of help are only a brief list of examples; sometimes we need more or different kinds of help. Sometimes the scope of the help we need is a more integrated approach, something more formal and tangible to help us access and stay present on our fulfillment path.

The social conditioning we've received says "I shouldn't need help, I should be strong enough to do what I need to do on my own". But if we can't receive, others can't successfully give. Learning to gracefully receive goes against our social conditioning, yet it is a crucial skill to learn. This social conditioning must be faced and disarmed as well, and in order to do that, we must face and release our shame and judgments about needing help and asking for help.

The Coffin Zone

Growth comes from taking risks and making changes. Staying more or less permanently in one's comfort zone makes it a "coffin zone". I do not want parts of me to become so deadened into routines and patterns that nothing ever shifts, as I slide inexorably into various levels of death. I try to keep swinging at something currently out of my reach, in order to continually infuse my life with vitality.

Transformation is possible, but not without major growth at all levels of our being. My path for the past thirty years has been one of constant change. I needed the stability of routines and known courses until I was thirty in order to have a "launching pad", and to see that the path I walked in those years is no longer my right path. I had to experience what I did not want in order to know for sure what I did want. I thank my parents for giving me the gift of a baseline level of stability for those first two-plus decades so that I could build the courage to make many eventual changes, not having burned out on changing constantly in childhood. Parts of me would like more comfort and stability now, but finding the right balance between comfort/stability and change can take time to fully manifest. There is nothing inherently wrong with comfort and stability as long as risky choices and refusal to compromise one's deepest desires and needs are added to the mix.

It occurs to me that I could well have titled this book, this process "Dealing and Healing". Finding a way to face head on to my past denials and ignorance, and using the tools I've found to take action to help myself live, seems to me like the 'dealing' part. Healing comes after dealing, right? Isn't healing the fruit of the labor?

But "Healing and Dealing" is the directionality that feels more right to me. Some subconscious part of me might have noticed then what I am aware of noticing now, in liking the chosen name – that healing is cyclical, like a spiral, and it never stops. We never stop ascending the spiral. We heal something, then from the new place we're in, we draw in the next experience or trigger, and then we deal again, and heal again, and on it goes. Somehow this point in the cycle, hard as it is, feels just a little easier somehow, overall, than "the last time I was here".

Our intention to heal is paramount, and initiatory. Without really intensely wanting to heal, or following through by dealing in each cycle, we start to die again, in many cases with regrets, with blame and feeling guilty, or via some heavy judgments on ourselves or "how the world is". We wall up in proportion to what degree, even subtly, we've given up.

Certainly this is not standard; human beings die in many states of being. Yet I feel intuitively that this sequence happens a lot across humanity. Those of you who have read this book sequentially to this point surely have a solid intent to heal and deal as fully as possible, no matter how much in denial you've been before, and we're all very, very good deniers. When I witness the healing intent of my fellow self-healers, I feel humbled and in admiration of the sacred pact within ourselves that we've made, to not stop, to just keep going, even if sometimes two steps forward, one back, or one step forward, two back.

Only you can know the changes you need to make. If you desire greater fulfillment you could ask your "deeper" or higher self to bring you visions of what your secret desires are, hidden from your conscious awareness. If you do get visions emanating from your buried desires, I wish for you the courage to reach for and manifest them.

Visions for Our New Life

'Chakra' is Sanskrit for 'wheel'. We all have seven major energy centers or chakras, vortices or wheels of energy located at key points from the tops of our heads to the bases of our spines. When a vision comes, it may come from one of two directions; descending from your topmost chakra at the crown of your head – or beginning deep in your root chakra and rising up towards your upper chakras. If it "grabs" you, it will pass through your heart chakra, the midpoint, where you will notice whether you love the vision or not. If you do love it, and want to give it life, it will travel on towards the remainder of your chakras to ground and manifest. In the process, it will run smack dab into your judgments and fears of why it cannot happen, could not possibly come true, all the reasons it is not a viable vision for you, etc.

We all have imbalances in various of our chakras. These blocks/imbalances make manifestations come out differently than we envisioned them. The imbalances stem from chronically repressing our emotional responses to various triggers, as well as being physical manifestations of denial such as ongoing addictive behaviors.

Bee Wolf-Ray suggests we help evolve and tune awareness of our chakras by cultivating a loose yet constant background sensory awareness of our crown's connection to Universal Chi, the inside of our heads, the back of our throat, our heartbeat or pulse, our diaphragm as we breathe, our belly, genitals and anus. If you try this, you may find a new, helpful habit forming, releasing any judgment that this awareness is not possible in the face of outward stimulation. You may find it quite triggering to do so, as engaging in this inner awareness may challenge numbness we habitually cultivate and awaken old feelings we didn't realize we had.

You may encounter frustration and fear as well as various other physical and emotional obstacles around making your visions come true, and perhaps find heartbreak that they have not happened already. You can allow those feelings to express to the best of your ability and acceptance, so that your beloved visions can manifest in a more evolved way. This evolution happens because emotional movement enables greater input from all parts of the Self into our dreams and visions. In doing so, you will be joining the healing and dealing tide rising on every shore of the planet.

Conclusion: Changing the World

"If you say you want a revolution, baby, well there's nothing like your own."
~ Karl Wallinger

I feel passionate about the spiritual homily, 'as without, so within'. If I reverse the words to read 'as within, so without', the meaning stands out in even bolder relief. Our collective inner state not only has huge impact on the outer state, it creates it, collectively.

"How the world is" is how our inner world is, and we are often blind to this fact because we cannot see directly into our "great subconscious" with our minds, which is by far, at this point in time, the largest part of our psyche, relative to the conscious part. Because it is larger, the subconscious has greater power to create our reality than the conscious. But because we do not know what is in our subconscious by its very definition as such, we cannot see how it is reflected by the outside world.

How To Make A Difference

Whether we dismiss it or act upon it, "how can I make a difference" is a question most of us challenge ourselves with whenever we hear of great injustice being played out on the world stage. Some of us choose to act, heading out to the front lines to face the oppressor.

Despite great courage and noble intent in doing so, we can ignore our inner state and our emotional habits, to our own great detriment and at cross-purposes to our agenda. When acting too soon or before we are really ready, in the midst of our honorable intent, we go past certain inner warnings. We then find ourselves suffering setbacks that, depending on their intensity, can throw us far enough off center that we either quit or are damaged in some way.

If I choose to act, it is vital to know that I am really aligned within first, among all my parts. I need to make sure I am not just responding to a loud, charged-up part of myself that has a lot of energy for a certain agenda.

The Impact of Personal Healing

I believe the most significant thing we can do is handle our fear, anger and grief differently than we always have. These three emotions make up the bulk of the unseen waters of the great and powerful subconscious. Release judgments that you cannot make a difference with an individual act of responsible emotional release, executed alone in a room.

Try it, if you have the slightest bit of curiosity as to whether releasing in such ways can work for you or help anything out there change. Sometimes the change is very gradual and subtle but that doesn't make it insignificant. Try it after you clamp down on your rising fear with words in your head telling you expressing fear in sound by yourself is stupid, useless or that you will just create more of it and never make it back out of it. Try it the next time your blood boils, and rage at the walls of an enclosed room in deafening sound instead of shouting words at your partner, your friend, your kids, your parents, or the authority figures inside the protest barrier. See what happens.

In so many of our lives, emotional expression is the one avenue we have not explored fully, with the intent to make meaningful change in our lives. When we express, we can meaningfully affect those whom we touch, and just maybe, the lives of those we have not even met.

"When you heal trauma, you heal the nervous system. When you heal the nervous system, you heal the emotional body. When you heal the emotional body, you heal the psychic (empathic) body. When you heal the psychic body, you heal the vibration. Once the vibration is healed, realities change."
~ Author Unknown

Accepting The Journey

The water runs dirty while the well is being cleaned. Sometimes we go through phases of feeling terrible amidst this process – these seasons come with the territory. There can be times where we are driven to go inside, to sit in the midst of our pain for a while and just be real with how we really feel before we are able to move enough of the pain, vibrate enough old denials to see more light than we were seeing before we dove into this latest layer.

A healing and dealing path of emotional expression is a pilgrimage, not a quick little 400 meter dash. It is an iterative, onion-peeling process. We will never be "all done" evolving our Selves at every level of being. All we can do is grow in acceptance of and resulting comfort with the journey we are all on.

Emotional backlog of lifetimes-long denial *is* finite, if huge, and if I change my question from "when will I be all done?" to "what is my responsibility in this situation?" I will end up a lot happier on the path and that much closer to true balance. After a while of building healing momentum, a passion for the process can develop.

We are becoming more sensitive on this path, not more impregnable, and we are becoming more emotional, not less. As we clear our backlog, however, the *tenor* of our process will change and emotional expression at all levels will eventually be as natural as breathing, a cry, yell, keen or scream as commonly heard, accepted and acceptable as a peal of laughter. Move it and move on.

Responsible expression of emotion is the one piece of the puzzle we have most potential access to and power to implement, the one piece most of us have never given a fair shake to see if it could actually help. Once we change our emotional habits of repression and blame, the outer world will never be the same. Do not be fooled by how long it takes, or how many times you have to repeat the process in order to make an inner or outer difference. Stevie Wonder spoke truth when he sang, "I say it's taking us so long, because we've got so far to come".

Welcome To The Revolution[2]

This one's for the revolution, a treeroots revolution
Welcome to the revolution, a treeroots revolution

A new day, where everyone plays
A new way, where we all have a say
A new list, where nobody's missed
A new twist, where we all get the gist

[2] *Milan Starcic contributed to this lyric*

288

This one's for the revolution, a treeroots revolution
Welcome to the revolution, a treeroots revolution

It's deeper than grass, and deep as the sea
It's really as deep as we want it to be
Deep in the Earth, welcome the Son
The Daughter, the Father, and The Mother as One
Deep into space, wide as the sky
Deep as our dreams we no longer deny
Deep in our pain, tears fall like rain
Healing and dealing again and again

This one's for the revolution, a treeroots revolution
Welcome to the revolution, a treeroots revolution

Changin' the preacher, changin' the prophet
Change what they've got for us on the docket
Changin' the rules, and changin' direction
Change the regime in the comin' election
Change into something just a little more strange
Changin' our fortunes into more than chump change
Change all the reasons why we've been cryin'
Change all the habits we've been denyin'

Changin' the tune, and changin' the flow
Let's change this world or She going to blow
I'll change me and you change you
I'll help you and you help me too
Change anything you're doing that's inflicting pain
Change nothing that's a-needin' to be left unchanged
Change thinkin' how you're thinkin' 'bout the opposite
sex
Getta change o' scenery, change your context

Change up the mood but stop changin' the food
Changin' the system so we'll never get sued
Change outta old clothes into the nude
Change being lewd she would rather be wooed

Change attitude, change it or we're screwed
Changin' the channel to that TV you're glued
Changin' the crude into something less rude
So Earth Changes don't crash into the 'hood!

This one's for the revolution, a treeroots revolution
Welcome to the revolution, a treeroots revolution

*　　*　　*　　*　　*　　*　　*　　*

Acknowledgements

To my partner Bee Wolf-Ray, the primary editor for Healing and Dealing: *Your brilliant, coherent and matter-of-fact syntheses of my ramblings made the articles which got expanded into this book even possible. Your ability to shoehorn my rough copy into 600 words every month was miraculous; I am as a child who never ceases to be amazed, not only that it fits but that I like it in the end! The fact that you live this stuff with me made the editing process exponentially easier, because you already knew what I meant. You are so gentle with me around this kind of writing, aware of the vulnerability inherent in the act. In addition to all the things I said in the Foreword, you have shaped my world-view and awareness in seminal ways.*

To my sister Alison Scannell, the conceptionist for the project: *Having been part of my long-winded dissertations on various healing topics, you suggested I make a book out of it. Without your enthusiastic encouragement and belief in my ability to unpack cans of worms like these, my monthly articles and this project would not even* have been begun. Kudos also for hanging in and dialoguing with me regarding some of these issues back in the day, which ultimately became several segments of this book.

To my mother Valerie Johnson: your thoughtful interactions, questions and open mind with regards to my non-mainstream take on healing gave me so much grist for the mill it made it possible to extend our email interactions into parts of this book, along with those I had with Alison and others, sewn together with my own ramblings.

To my father Alan Johnson for helping emphasize the finer points of the English language all my life, encouraging me to write, and supporting my gifts the ways you did, emotionally and financially.

To Bee Wolf-Ray, Seamas Manly, Nathalie St. Amant, Sara-Mandal Joy, Kendra Thomas, Robert Dagostino and Jean Gordy for your willingness to contribute segments for publication that aligned so seamlessly with my material.

To the volunteers on the staff of the HI First Edition, in particular editors Reina LeBaron, Judy Goffman, Jenny Brown, Ken Clark and Cat Dextrase: your willingness to publish me every month between 2003-07 gave me the confidence I needed. I also feel grateful to the paper for the monthly deadline, as it has encouraged me to write, where writing may not have happened at all otherwise in any kind of regular or timely way.

To both the First Ed and Healing and Dealing blog readerships who fed back: the additional confidence boost and confirmation that I was on the right track was important and necessary rocket fuel.

To my editing team: Bee Wolf-Ray, Su Carson, Nathalie St-Amant, Dawn Tirschel and Seamas Manly for responding to my repeated callouts over time and offering much needed feedback and edits — the book is a way better and cleaner read for having been gone over so carefully and skillfully by each of you.

To freelance editor Leah Albrecht: Your offer and time taken to assist me in overhauling and finalizing the structural integrity of this book, in ways I didn't even realize I needed got me to the finish line in a very professional and skillful manner.

To Christine Torres for suggesting the outline of this book by posting my first fifteen articles gratis in five sections on her website so I could have some web presence for this material early on, side by side with her own very complementary and crucial healing writings.

("The Pathway Home:"
http://cyquest.abathyr.com/pathway/index.html)

To the many movers who received me over time, especially in email: you gave me the opportunity to witness my own understandings in front of me where I could see them, and helped me shape them with your own.

To Ceanne DeRohan for the great gift of your inspirational work; you are the grandmother of this book.

To Loving Mother and Father, in all forms and non-forms Physical, Emotional, Mental, and Spiritual: this book wouldn't exist without Your guidance and support.

Related Reading

There are some outstanding articles, essays, fiction and links on emotional expression and attitudes about emotions written by a friend (and her mother) who have been expressing their emotions since 1967. I find the writing on this vintage website really accessible, clear, and free of jargon:
http://cyquest.abathyr.com/

The author of this site has a body of work that comprises some of my main source material. She has brought forth a number of books on the kind of emotional healing and dealing that I feel is crucial in these times. The FAQ page on the website I find particularly clear and informative.
http://www.rightuseofwill.com

A bodyworker who gets it on the emotional level:
https://myofascialtrainings.com/working-emotional-release-awareness-bodywork-sessions/

A brilliant writer, compassionate, knowledgeable and embodying the loving masculine:
https://www.goodreads.com/author/quotes/434 0155.Jeff_Brown

Some excellent suggestions on how to allow old emotions up to the surface and release them:
https://theglobalsuccessacademy.com/all-subconscious-blockages-are-repressed-emotions/

Short, excellent "healing and dealing" style approach to emotional release:
http://joy2meu.com/emotions.html

For those who feel ready to take the red pill into the depths:
https://finalresponsibility.wordpress.com/about -beearthing/

About The Author

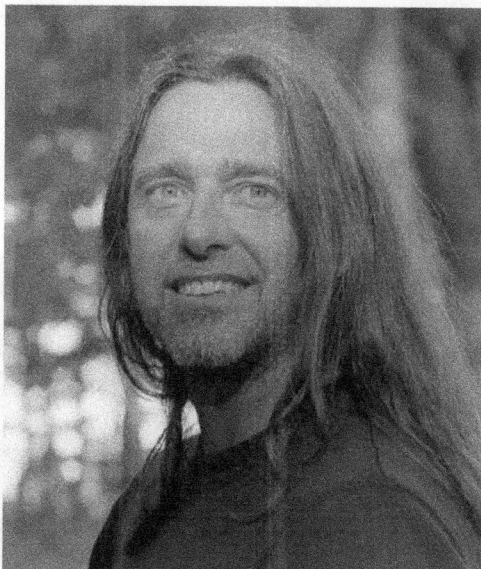

photo credit: Melissa Moore

Peter Cloud Panjoyah is a healing facilitator
  whose main client is himself. He is also a lover,
  father, poet, mover, songwriter, musician,
  astrologer, life coach, masseur, entrepreneur
  and radio DJ. In a past life he obtained a B.A. in
  English and American Literature and Language
  at Harvard University. "Healing and Dealing" is
  his first book. He lives in the Gulf Islands of
  British Columbia and welcomes readers to
  contact him or leave feedback via his webpage,
  https://healinganddealing.net

www.ingramcontent.com/pod-product-compliance
Lightning Source LLC
Chambersburg PA
CBHW020525270326
41927CB00006B/450